# The Social World of Older People

*by Christina Victor, Sasha Scambler and John Bond*

Open University Press

Open University Press
McGraw-Hill Education
McGraw-Hill House
Shoppenhangers Road
Maidenhead
Berkshire
England
SL6 2QL
email: enquiries@openup.co.uk
world wide web: www.openup.co.uk

and Two Penn Plaza, New York, NY 10121-2289, USA

First published 2009

A catalogue record of this book is available from the British Library

ISBN-10: 0-335-21521-1 pb, 0-335-21522-X hb
ISBN-13: 978-0-335-21521-8 pb, 978-0-335-21522-5 hb
1005695719

Library of Congress Cataloging-in-Publication Data
CIP data applied for

Typeset by YHT Ltd, London
Printed in Great Britain by Bell & Bain Ltd, Glasgow

# The Social World of
# Older People

**Growing Older**

Series Editor: Alan Walker

The objective of this series is to showcase the major outputs from the ESRC Growing Older programme and to provide research insights which will result in improved understanding and practice and enhanced and extended quality of life for older people.

It is well known that people are living longer but until now very little attention has been given to the factors that determine the quality of life experienced by older people. This important new series will be vital reading for a broad audience of policymakers, social gerontologists, social policy analysists, nurses, social workers, sociologists and social geographers as well as advanced undergraduate and postgraduate students in these disciplines.

**Series titles include:**

Ann Bowling *Ageing Well*

Joanne Cook, Tony Maltby and Lorna Warren *Older Women's Lives*

Mary Maynard, Haleh Afshar, Myfanwy Franks and Sharon Wray *Women in Later Life*

Sheila Peace, Caroline Holland and Leonie Kellaher *Environment and Identity in Later Life*

Thomas Scharf, Chris Phillipson and Allison E. Smith *Ageing in the City*

Christina Victor, Sasha Scambler and John Bond *The Social World of Older People*

Alan Walker (ed.) *Growing Older in Europe*

Alan Walker and Catherine Hagan Hennessy (eds) *Growing Older: Quality of Life in Old Age*

Alan Walker (ed.) *Understanding Quality of Life in Old Age*

# Contents

# Preface and acknowledgements

This book is the culmination of a research project that was funded as part of the ESRC Growing Older Programme. When we first decided to collaborate with our colleague Ann Bowling on a number of grant applications to the Growing Older Programme we did not anticipate the germ of an idea that we should revisit ideas about loneliness in social isolation would rouse the imagination of the commissioning panel. That it did pleasantly surprised us. At the outset we were concerned by the way ideas about loneliness and social isolation were contributing to the negative stereotypes of later life and underpinning of ageism. We wanted to re-evaluate the place of loneliness and social isolation in social gerontological literature and argue for a more parsimonious use of the concept in policy and practice. To do this we needed to ground our critical arguments in the evidence of new data about contemporary social relations in later life. The Growing Older Programme gave us the space to reflect on these important ideas and collect the new survey and qualitative interview data that we needed to execute our research agenda.

The research was funded by the Economic and Social Research Council (ESRC) as part of the Growing Older Programme (Award No. L480254042 [Loneliness and social isolation]). The survey was part funded by grants held collaboratively by Professor Ann Bowling, Professor Stephen Sutton and Dr David Banister (ESRC Award No. L480254003 [Quality of Life]) and Professor Shah Ebrahim (MRC Health Service Research Collaboration Award No. NNN [Health and Disability]).

We are grateful to the Office of National Statistics (ONS) Omnibus Survey staff, and the ONS Qualitative Research Unit, in particular Maureen Kelly, Olwen Rowlands, Jack Eldridge and Kirsty Deacon for their much appreciated advice and help with designing the main questionnaire, for conducting focus groups with older people to inform the design of the questionnaire, for sampling and overseeing the 'Quality of Life Interview' and processing the data. We would like to thank the ONS interviewers, Professor Janet Peacock and Louise

Marston for statistical advice and Cath Brennand, and Cheryl Wiscombe who assisted in the preparation of the manuscript. We are also grateful to Professor Ann Bowling who was a co-applicant of the ESRC grant (Award No. .L48025404).

Those who carried out the original analysis and collection of survey data hold no responsibility for the further analysis and its interpretation. Material from the ONS Omnibus Survey, made available through ONS, has been used with the permission of the controller of the Stationary Office. The ONS Omnibus dataset was deposited by ONS on the Data Archive at the University of Essex; the qualitative data was deposited by the research team on the Qualitative Data Archive also at the University of Essex. We are also grateful to Cambridge University (Ageing and Society; Reviews in Clinical Gerontology; Social Policy and Society), Pavilion (Quality and Ageing) and the editors Professor Alan Walker and Catherine Hagan Hennessy and Open University Press for permission to use already published material.

Finally we especially would like to thank all those older people who gave so freely of their time to participate in this study. Without them this book would not have been possible.

## Publications stemming from the research

Victor, C., Scambler, S., Bond, J. and Bowling, A. (2000) 'Being alone in later life: loneliness, social isolation and living alone', *Reviews in Clinical Gerontology*, 10, pp. 407-417.

Victor, C., Scambler, S., Bond, J. and Bowling, A. (2002a) 'Loneliness in later life: preliminary findings from the Growing Older project', *Quality in Ageing*, 3, (1), pp. 34-41.

Victor, C. R., Scambler, S. J., Bond, J. and Bowling, A. (2004) 'Loneliness in later life', in Walker, A. and Hennessy, C. H.(eds) *Growing older: quality of life in old age*. Open University Press: Maidenhead, pp. 107-126.

Victor, C. R., Scambler, S. J., Bowling, A. and Bond, J. (2005a) 'The prevalence of, and risk factors for, loneliness in later life: a survey of older people in Great Britain', *Ageing and Society*, 25, (3), pp. 357-376.

Victor, C. R., Scambler, S. J., Marston, L., Bond, J. and Bowling, A. (2005b) 'Older people's experiences of loneliness in the UK: does gender matter?' *Social Policy and Society*, 5, (1), pp. 27-38.

Victor, C. R., Scambler, S. J., Shah, S., Cook, D. G., Harris, T., Rink, E. and de Wilde, S. (2002b) 'Has loneliness amongst older people increased? An investigation into variations between cohorts', *Ageing and Society*, 22, (5), pp. 585-597.

Victor, C. R. and Scharf, T. (2005) 'Social isolation and loneliness', in Walker, A.(ed), *Understanding quality of life in old age*. Open University Press: Maidenhead, pp. 100-116.

# 1

# Introduction

At the beginning of a new millennium social worlds are changing. Developments in the physical environment, scientific and technological innovation, the reorganisation of work and leisure and the impact of globalisation and global capitalism have varyingly influenced the nature of the world in which we now live. Social engagement and relationships, however, remain important at any age and their quality is a key element contributing to the quality of life of older people (Bond and Corner, 2004; Bowling, 2005). Framed by networks of kin and friends, participation in activities and hobbies, the enactment of social roles and the nature of social relationships is shaped and modified by experiences along the life course through the dynamic interaction of time and place.

Contemporary stereotypes of social engagement and relationships in later life remain essentially negative reinforced over the past 60 years by the focus in British gerontology on the problems of old age (McIntyre, 1977) and highlighted in public policy. 'Loneliness' and 'social isolation' have been part of social gerontological policy and public discourses since the development of the Welfare State in 1948. The two concepts are often conflated and used interchangeably by gerontologists, policymakers and the wider public. The purpose of this book is to challenge these negative discourses by critically reviewing our understandings of loneliness and social isolation through the accounts of older people and through the modelling of their likely causes. This is not to deny the existence of loneliness or social isolation in later life but rather to show that they have always been a minority experience and are not an inevitable part of 'normal' ageing. We argue that loneliness and social isolation are experienced at all stages of the life course and are not unique to the social world of older people. Our goal is to highlight the positive experience of later life and those factors that protect older people against the vicissitudes of loneliness and social isolation.

In recent years the importance of social relationships and social participation in later life has been reflected in the emerging policy rhetoric of social inclusion and social exclusion (Office of the Deputy Prime Minister, 2006). Initially, the social inclusion/exclusion agenda had been driven by concerns about the integration of disadvantaged families and young people who were unemployed. Across the life course social inclusion and social exclusion have been defined in terms of access to social engagement and participation. These include access to social relationships through family and friendship networks; access to cultural activities (e.g. bingo halls and cinemas); access to civic activities (e.g. membership of local religious, voluntary or leisure-based organisations); access to local services; and access to financial resources. In an attempt to address ageism, this policy rhetoric has started to highlight the importance of enabling older people (and younger people) to have meaningful social roles and to participate more widely in society. Through greater social engagement older citizens will develop social capital for themselves, their families and their communities. Whilst we do not share all the tenets of the social inclusion/exclusion policy discourse that engages the attention of national and local government, many of these ideas provide a useful organising framework and policy context for the material covered within this book. However, 'loneliness' and 'social isolation' within the broader context of social engagement and social relationships remain our focus.

## Social relationships and quality of life

There already exists an established literature on quality of life and older people (see Bond and Corner, 2004; Bowling, 2005) and we do not propose to provide yet another review. A number of key themes emerge from this literature that indicate a need to examine further social relationships and social engagement in later life. Much of this literature focuses on defining quality of life for older people and how quality of life is operationalised and measured. On this topic there are also a number of empirical studies that demonstrate how quality of life varies within the older population, what factors promote or inhibit quality of life and how quality of life in later life differs (or not) from other phases of the life course (see Farquhar, 1994; Bowling et al., 2002; Bajekal et al., 2004; Blane et al., 2004; Bond and Corner, 2004; Gabriel and Bowling, 2004a and 2004b; Moriarty and Butt, 2004; Nazroo et al., 2004; Smith et al., 2004; Walker and Hennessy, 2004; Bowling, 2005; Higgs et al., 2005; Holland et al., 2005; Scharf et al., 2005b; Walker, 2005). In many of these studies social relations and social engagement are both seen as one of a number of components of quality of life along with other components such as the environment, health status and access to material resources. Social relations and social engagement do not form the focus of attention but rather are of interest as explanatory concepts for the wider understanding of quality of life. Much of the theoretical work within the quality of life tradition has been heavily influenced by psychological perspectives, focusing upon individual factors with an emphasis on measurement issues and the search for statistical associations and predictions (see Bond and Corner, 2004; Bowling, 2005). Along with Bond and Corner (2004) we would argue that the social and sociological context is often missing from such empirical work and that there is a need to develop a perspective where social relations are a key focus. This is the aspect of quality of life and ageing that we are seeking to address.

## Social engagement and social capital

The work investigating 'social capital' is another illustration of the large body of empirical and theoretical work which, whilst more obviously focusing upon social engagement, provides only a partial perspective upon the social world of older people (and indeed other age groups). The field of research investigating the definition and measurement of 'social capital' is extensive and there is a broad distinction to be drawn between the economic and sociological approaches. The more sociological approaches seek to quantify individual social relationships, support mechanisms and access to 'social resources'. This latter element often forms the prime focus of such studies as the emphasis in much social-capital-related work is upon understanding how social resources can be mobilised in times of 'need'. Here, again, there are subtle but important differences in the emphases between work within this tradition and our work. With an explicit focus upon accessing social resources to respond to (informal) care needs there is a tendency to 'problematise' older peoples' social relationships as 'resources' available to provide support and care in times of crisis. We can contrast this approach with our interests in understanding the extent, nature and meaning of such relationships for their own sake rather than as resources to be accessed (or indeed as contributors of help to others' problems). As with many other aspects of the study of later life there is an emphasis in some work concerned with family relationships to 'pathologising' everyday experiences and activities of older people. To overstate our case, friendship and kinship ties are only seen to be of interest to researchers as potential resources in times of crisis, with the emphasis upon how groups contribute to the support of older people (rather than vice versa) rather than being important in their own right. This illustrates a recurrent theme within British social gerontological research, which is to focus upon the 'problematic' aspects of old age and later life and to problematise 'normal' aspects of the daily life of older people such as kinship and friendship networks and engagement in 'normal' social activities.

## Social relations and social engagement in later life

In this book our focus is upon describing and understanding the social world of older people in terms of social relations and social engagement. Loneliness and social isolation are our primary foci. We take as the exemplar of our approach the pioneering work of Townsend (1957) in his study of *The Family Life of Old People* based in the post-war East End of London and work by other authors such as Rosser and Harris (1965) in their study of social relationships in post-war Swansea. We argue that our book complements the extensive body of existing literature on quality of life in later life, literature which provides only a partial gaze upon social relationships and social engagement. We take an explicitly sociological rather than psychological approach because we consider that the study of social relationships is much broader than that demonstrated by much contemporary quality-of-life research. The outcomes from psychologically orientated quality-of-life research and policy research that focuses on 'caring' aspects of social relationships needs to be located within a much broader social context. Similarly, whilst the problematic dimensions of relationships in later life such as exclusion, isolation and loneliness are important, we argue that these can only properly be understood by locating them within the broader context of social relationships. However, we are not seeking to directly reproduce the work of Townsend (1957), since in part this has already been done by Phillipson and colleagues (2001b). Rather it is the theoretical approach and in the primary focus of our book on social relationships that we see our link with Townsend (1957) and other community studies of that era (Young and Willmott, 1957; Marris, 1958; Rosser and Harris, 1965; Tunstall, 1966).

Our book reflects the many changes in the nature of society and social ties that have characterised Britain since these early studies and we draw a wider boundary around social relationships than the focus upon family and kinship. When thinking about the composition of the social world of older people there is an almost inevitable focus upon family and kinship groups. The title of Townsend's book, *The Family Life of Old People*, encapsulates society's implicit assumptions about older people's patterns of social engagement. Examining the contents page of his book demonstrates the focus upon primary kinship links and close relationships such as spouse, children and siblings. This probably reflects the concern to document the availability of potential informal carers to support older people in times of crisis as well as reflecting the very different social context that characterised Britain in the decade after the establishment of the Welfare State. Less emphasis was given to understanding the broader social context in which older people were located, how this was maintained, how this represented a continuation or discontinuity with earlier phases of life and how relationships were mediated within a spatial context. This preoccupation within both the family sociology and social gerontology traditions with changes in the structure, and by implication, nature and role of families in the lives of older people, continued to the millenium. In this book we focus upon the wider social environment as suggested by Phillipson et al. (2001) and Phillipson (2007) as this provides the context within which most of us enact our lives. Like them we argue that the experience of growing older is shaped by the broader social context which includes family and kinship groups but also encompasses wider social relationships such as friends and neighbours and relationships based upon specific roles and functions such as work or recreational-based relationships. As Askham and colleagues (2007) have recently argued, social relationships in later life are not just about family and kinship. We also suggest that socio-structural factors such as class, gender and ethnicity operate to influence and contextualise social engagement and that these factors have not been given the emphasis that their influence over other aspects of later life such as health, access to services and access to financial and other resources would suggest that they merit.

Implicit in this introduction is the notion that there are two distinct, but related, types of research questions that we can ask about social relationships in later life. First, we can identify a suite of usually quantitative questions concerned with establishing the frequency of contact between different groups of individuals, the size and composition of an individual's social network, and the activities that individuals participate in. However, there is a second and equally important series of questions that relate to how individuals evaluate the quality of their social relationships, the activities that they engage in, and the nature and meaning of notions such as isolation, exclusion and loneliness. In order to provide a comprehensive examination of this topic we argue that both sets of issues require addressing and we attempt to undertake that in this book. However, these questions derive from different research paradigms and, as such, require specific but linked types of research methods, data collection and data analysis. We use two major primary datasets to examine this topic, which are described in detail in the next chapter, and we, where possible, adopt a life-course approach and examine relationships from this perspective. As such this is a 'mixed methods' study that aims to start to unravel the complexity of older peoples' social relationships by employing two major approaches to data collection – a large quantitative survey and a substantial series of qualitative 'in-depth' interviews.

Older people are not immune from social change. They experience this along with other groups within the population. Whilst our data relate to a specific temporal context – approximately the turn of the millennium – where possible, we locate our empirical material within a broader socio-historical context to attempt to establish the continuities and changes in the social world of older people and how this differs from that experienced by their counterparts 50 years ago as documented in the works of Sheldon (1948), Townsend (1957), Tunstall (1966), Rosser and Harris (1965) and Young and Willmott (1957). These classic studies often examined social relationships within specific geographical contexts such as the Bethnal Green district of London. As such they are often referred to as 'community studies'. The epithet 'classic' is testimony to the importance and longevity of the material that these researchers collected, the methodological approaches they employed and for the influence they had upon the development of social research at that time. These texts offer us the opportunity to develop an explicitly comparative perspective to our work and to start to unravel and document the changes in the experience of old age over time.

There is an inherent tendency within much academic research to focus upon specific countries and cultures, especially when such research is driven by nationally defined social and welfare policy concerns. However, as well as trying to include a temporal dimension within our research, we also use comparative material from other countries where available, again to try to determine how the experience of older people in Britain reflects those of their contemporaries in other Western industrial countries. Whilst there is a large culturally and socially defined dimension to the experience of social relationships in later life, we feel that there is much to be gained in our understanding of ageing and later life by adopting an international perspective. By drawing explicit comparisons with previous points in our own history and with other societies, we can start to tease out the continuities in the way that older people experience and describe their social relationships and what the elements that vary culturally and historically are.

In the rest of this chapter we outline the broad context that forms the social world of older people, introduce key terms, describe our broad methodological approach and outline the aims and background to our study. In Chapter 2 we provide an overview of the theoretical underpinning of research concerned with loneliness and isolation, provide a summary of our methods and measures, and provide broad details of the nature and characteristics of the people included within the study that forms the basis of this book. In our three empirically based chapters we focus upon presenting the meaning and patterns of older people's social relationships, using both quantitative and qualitative data, and in our final chapter we consider the implications for theory, policy and practice.

# The social world of older people

What activities, links and relationships form the social world of older people? How do these relationships, activities and ties ebb and flow across the life course? How are they influenced by the socio-spatial context within which older people live? How, if at all, do they change over the life course and vary within and between different cohorts of older people? How does the pattern and web of relationships demonstrated by older people differ from those for people from differing age groups? How do the experiences of social engagement and social relationships vary between different countries? These core questions are at the heart of our research and underpin the arguments and evidence presented in this book.

The experience of ageing, and other components of the life course such as adolescence, takes place within a powerful framework of the family and wider social relationships. As we move through the life course we belong to a dynamic set of kinship and socially defined groups, which bring engagement and interaction with work colleagues, family, friends and neighbours and those with whom we share common interests and beliefs. These often reside within a common geographical space such as a neighbourhood, village or town or, more recently, notions of 'virtual' communities linked by the internet and world wide web. In addition, there are also social links with 'formally' based social groups such as statutory agencies providing health or social care services or voluntary agencies, which need to be factored in to our analysis of older people's social engagement. These groups, and our relationships with them, wax and wane across the life course as family dynamics, friendship networks and work or leisure-based relationships evolve in response to changes in our social circumstances and geographical mobility.

This description is neither unique to older people nor to Britain nor to this specific temporal context. However, our knowledge of the social world and social relationships remains partial as much of the research either treats social relationships as a 'secondary' variable to be used to 'explain' some other feature of interest such as overall quality of life, or the perspective is very firmly fixed upon the function of social relationships in the provision of care or support in times of crisis such as bereavement or major illness. Research in Britain has predominantly focused upon studying caring for people. The focus has been on the provision of help with instrumental activities of daily living – activities labelled by Parker (1985) as 'tending' – rather than understanding the emotional and social roots of such relationships. Similarly, in studying social relationships, the focus in previous research has been largely upon the 'pathological' aspects such as loneliness and isolation and with providing complex typologies of networks. Much less interest has been shown in understanding the meaning of such relationships and how they are mediated and shaped by both the broad socio-spatial context and the personal biographies and experiences of the protagonists.

The degree to which older people are embedded within a network of social relationships framed around kin, friends, colleagues and neighbours provides a context and a framework within which ageing is experienced. We readily acknowledge that such relationships provide a major resource base with which to negotiate the challenges that ageing can pose. In this broad sense older people are no different from other age groups where family, friends and colleagues help us to navigate the events that we may experience across the life course, such as relationship breakdown, major illness or financial problems, and more positive changes, such as marriage, moving into a new house or flat and the birth and raising of children. Clearly those people that we turn to in times of crisis are those we also choose to celebrate our good fortune and achievements, with both personal and professional relationships. We acknowledge that social relationships in later life are more than just a prelude to the provision of care. We also believe that studies of social exchange within and between families are very valuable for revealing the dynamic and life-course component of many relationships, especially those that are kin based. It is part, if not all, of this broader framework of engagement that we are seeking to expose to view in this book.

The specific interests of researchers studying the social relationships of older people shows considerable variation over time, as does the centrality of their focus upon social relationships. This reflects the interrelationship between the maturing of our discipline as an area of academic activity, the interests of researchers from a variety of different academic disciplines and the developing policy agenda. We should not under-estimate the importance of our medical colleagues in identifying the significance of social relations to the quality of life and well-being of older people. For example, Sheldon's study of Wolverhampton, perhaps not surprisingly as the author was a pioneering geriatrician, focused upon the medical aspects of later life. However, he did attempt to include a social element and he looked at help received from the family and also included a question on loneliness which was both novel and demonstrated a concern for social well-being that characterised many of the pioneering geriatricians such as Lionel Cosin and Marjorie Warren. A similar concern is demonstrated by the work of Bernard Isaacs – a geriatrician working in Glasgow (Isaacs et al., 1972).

The initial studies of Townsend (1957) and Rosser and Harris (1965) focused upon understanding relationships within and between households within a specific spatial context: the East End of London and Swansea, respectively. More recently, feminist-inspired scholars have been concerned with examining the gendered nature of the provision of 'informal' family-based care to frail older people (Finch, 1989; Finch and Groves, 1983; Graham, 1983), rather than with a wider perspective upon the social relationships of older people. Researchers such as Tunstall (1966) focused upon the 'pathological' or problematic aspects of social relationships. It is clear from the data generated from these various studies that there were a group of highly active and engaged older people. Yet, this is passed over and is not remarked on because of the focus upon the 'problems' of old age. More recently, Scharf and colleagues (2001) have focused upon 'social exclusion'. Hence research in this area of gerontology, like other aspects of our discipline, reflects the fashions and interests of researchers and the concerns of policy makers and practitioners as the recent interest in social exclusion testifies (Office of the Deputy Prime Minister, 2006), as well as an emphasis upon the negative or problematic aspects of social relationships in later life.

In understanding the social embeddedness of older people, both the availability of, and quality of, relationships with family and wider social relationships are important. To fully understand this topic we need to consider both the extent and degree of social involvement and the meaning of such relationships. Hence this is a research topic which benefits from the integration of both quantitative and qualitative methods. The meaning and value attached by individuals to specific forms of social contact varies and we might speculate that there is not a perfect fit between the quantity and quality of social relationships. So we may have strong close relationships with people we see or talk to only rarely or, conversely, not value especially highly the relationships with people or organisations with whom we have frequent dealings. Understanding such conundrums and apparent contradictions calls for an approach which focuses upon understanding the meaning of relationships as much as quantifying the number and amounts of relationships and suggests that we need to locate such linkages within a life-course context. Hence we are trying to provide an overview which can, at least partially, address such complex questions.

In this book we argue for the revival of the explicitly sociological contribution to the analysis of older people's social worlds. We are concerned with the broad topic of the engagement between older people and the wider society and how this is influenced by key social variables such as gender, class, ethnicity and age. This was the approach pioneered by Townsend (1957, 1973 and with Tunstall, 1968) and is evident in his comparative studies with Ethel Shanas (1968). Over the intervening four decades the study of social relationships in later life has become dominated by studies emphasising psychological aspects, health status, mental well-being and benefits of social relationships rather than issues of broader 'social meaning' and understanding of the 'social world' from the older person's perspective. Social relationships have been seen as independent variables explaining dependent variables such as psychological well-being, physical health or mental health rather than being important in their own right. Whilst important the psychological and mental health focus provides only a partial perspective upon what is a very complex multi-faceted phenomenon. Furthermore, the focus in such studies is often upon providing explanations at the level of the individual rather than drawing links with social structures, social institutions, place and social groups or examining the variation in patterns of social engagement within the differing sub-groups of the older population such as gender, class or ethnicity.

There has also been a large body of work generated by social policy concerns with 'population ageing' and influenced in varying degrees by notions of 'apocalyptic demography' (Robertson, 1997). In particular, the implications of contemporary demographic trends for the current (and future) availability of family and friends to provide 'informal' care to older people in the community has generated a large body of work documenting who provides care to older people, how much care is provided and what types of care are provided. Although useful in exposing to public gaze the contribution of women (and men) to the care of older people, the driving force behind such work is, at least in part, the auditing of the 'replacement costs' of the unpaid labour provided by family and friends. This presents only a partial gaze upon the social context within which older people are located and it is distorted by the emphasis upon care and the provision of care and a focus on the current pattern of linkages without attempting to locate them within a broader social context or to understand how such patterns have evolved. Clearly the results of such projects offer a distorted view on social links by the heavy focus upon the need for and provision of care. Such a perspective also excludes the broader social inclusion agenda by not including important social roles such as civic activities, volunteering and broader cultural participation.

Notions of social engagement are much broader than the narrow focus generated by either of the above two approaches. In this book we aim to redress the balance by offering a more expansive perspective rooted within an approach that emphasises the link between older people and the broader society. We include, in varying degrees of depth, the differing aspects of social engagement including: social relationships (contact with family and friends); cultural activities (visits to cinema, theatre, concerts, etc.); civic-based activities (membership of local groups/organisations, volunteering and voting) combined with access to basic services (health/social care services plus shops); neighbourhood; access to financial resources and consumption of material goods (holidays and household utilities, consumer goods, etc.). These link back to the conceptualisation of social inclusion/exclusion proposed by Scharf and colleagues (2001) and described in the report of the Office of the Deputy Prime Minister (2006).

However, these aspects of social life of older people do not remain constant. All of these dimensions are influenced by the constantly changing wider social context. An example of the importance of this in understanding the social relationships of older people is provided by Jerrome's (1993) analysis of the social factors influencing family relationships; factors that continue to exert an influence upon the social world that we all inhabit. Leaving aside for the moment the difficult issue of what specifically defines 'a family', she argues that five sets of social factors are influential in informing the family relationships of older people and, we would argue, by extension to the wider social topic of social engagement.

First, the well-documented demographic changes which have characterised Britain over the past hundred years, increasing longevity and reduced family sizes, have profoundly influenced the size and age distribution of families. Hence there is an increase in the number of family groups covering four, five or even six generations whilst the number of people within each generational tier is decreased. Given the primacy of the family in all of our social relationships, changes in family sizes inevitably influence the subsequent relationships.

Second, changes in the role of women in society, especially in the field of employment and educational opportunities, have altered gender relationships within the wider society. Women, who in previous cohorts would have looked predominantly to kin or neighbourhood for their social focus, now participate more widely within the work context which offers another arena for developing social relationships and ties.

Third, legislative changes, especially regarding issues such as the availability of divorce, access to abortion and equal opportunities legislation all influence the nature and structure of families and family-based relationships. For example, the availability of divorce as a means of ending unsatisfactory marriage combined with remarriage has resulted in the creation of 'blended' families. Although by no means novel or unique to contemporary society, like single-parent families, such forms of family structures are more common than in previous times. The complexity of such family groups requires the negotiation of new sets of social roles, relationships and responsibilities. Similarly co-habitation and civil partnerships demonstrate the constantly evolving form of what may broadly be defined as family groups and relationships.

Changes in social attitudes and ideology have altered many of our expectations of what is 'expected' or what the social norms are regarding family formation, expectations of marriage and parenthood and the new roles of great (and even great great) grandparents, aunts and uncles. For example, the availability of contraception and abortion has influenced the number of women having children, the timing of such offspring or if, indeed, they have any children at all. The work of Evandrou and Falkingham (2000) has drawn attention to the variations between cohorts in the numbers of women remaining childless. If the percentage of women remaining childless remains at the 20 per cent reported at age 40 for the 1960 cohort, there will be entering old age in the 2020s, groups of elders who do not have access to the kin networks of current groups. Furthermore, if the reduction in family size remains constant, then people in this cohort are also unlikely to be members of extended families. This presents a very different family context within which to experience old age in comparison to 50 years ago as described by Townsend (1957).

Finally, but perhaps more speculatively, rising levels of economic prosperity and the provision of welfare benefits have served to loosen the economic ties within families. In contemporary Western societies older people are not, as a result of the creation of pensions and welfare infrastructure, generally, directly economically dependent upon younger members of their families, although there are obvious financial co-dependencies across the generations. Taken in combination these factors have served to shape the nature of families and hence directly influence one of the arenas within which older people engage.

## Social networks and social support

The social networks of older people provide the keystone to understanding their social world. Researchers, not solely from the field of gerontology, have expended considerable intellectual activity and energy in the definition and analysis of social networks and establishing the links with health, disease and quality of life across a variety of different populations (see Phillipson et al., 2004). Indeed the term 'social network' has wide currency as it is used both within a social research context and more popular discourse. However, the frequency with which the term is used in research, lay and policy discourses renders it vulnerable to 'terminological inexactitute' in a fashion similar to other popularly used concepts such as community care. It can mean all things to all men and women. At the most superficial level the term 'social network' refers to the web or network of relationships within which, in our case, an older person is situated. Such networks may, or may not, be spatially defined. Hence social network represent the 'accumulation' of relationships and interactions across a variety of settings both social (family, friends or groups) or places (village, workplace). As such networks are seen as a key component or building block of the concept of social capital, at least from the sociological perspective.

Within this apparently straightforward concept there are a number of different aspects of social networks which are not always made explicit. At their most basic social networks identify and define the relationships associated with a specific individual. Relationships within social networks may be based around kinship or friendship ties, neighbourhood co-location or professional-based care (or other service-related) linkages. The status of service providers, either directly employed by the older person or provided via state agencies, is especially problematic within the context of network studies. However, defining what is, and is not, a relationship is far from straightforward. They are the foundation for the structural basis for networks and are clearly central to the empirical measurement of networks. Indeed the whole measurement dimension of social networks remains contentious with concepts such as 'network' poorly operationalised, with no clarity of the underlying theoretical concepts and with doubts and uncertainty as to the psychometric properties of measures.

A key distinction is made between social networks and social support. Social support refers to the provision of financial, instrumental or emotional support from network members (Bowling et al., 1989; Bowling and Browne, 1991) and so is focused upon the behavioural component of networks. Langford et al. (1997) identify the four main types of social support as: emotional, instrumental, informational and appraisal. They note that social networks and social embeddness are the precursors of support. Whilst not all members of the network may be called upon to provide support, it is highly unlikely that those outside of the network will be asked to do so. Hence the social network circumscribes the maximum boundaries of support theoretically available to an individual at a given point in time. There is within this definition, however, a presumption of support as flowing one way – from network members to the older person – rarely is the focus upon understanding what the older person has contributed (or is currently providing) to network members.

The definition and analysis of older people's social networks has formed an important and enduring strand within European (Lubben et al., 2006), American (Antonucci and Akiyama, 1987; Antonucci, 1990; Antonucci, 2001) and British gerontological research. Townsend (1957), Wenger (1984), Bowling et al. (1991) and Phillipson et al. (2001) have all undertaken substantive studies of social relationships in later life. The capturing and quantifying of participants' social networks has formed an important aspect of these authors' work. Phillipson and colleagues (Phillipson et al., 2001) undertook a 'restudy' of the neighbourhoods of Wolverhampton, the East End of London and Woodford Green, replicating the work of Sheldon (1948), Townsend (1957) and Young and Willmott (1957), respectively. They report that, for their samples, the average social network consisted of 9.3 people; women have larger networks than men (10.1 versus 8.2) but there was no obvious relationship with age. Wenger (1984), in her study in North Wales, reported that 25 per cent of her respondents had a network consisting of five or less persons.

Within the UK perhaps the most well-known researcher in the area of social support and social networks for older people is Clare Wenger (Wenger, 1991; Wenger and St Leger, 1992; Wenger et al., 2002). Drawing upon this research she has developed a network typology (see Chapter 5) based upon data collected about older people's kinship structure; contact with family members, friends and neighbours; and the level of participation in community and voluntary groups within a small area in North Wales. This is, of course, very similar data to that which has been collected in community surveys about the frequency of social contact. The estimation of social contact frequency plays an important role in the determination of the five network types. The network types are characterised by names that reflect the nature of the relationship the older person (ego) has to the social network. Three of the five types emphasise the importance of local kin, while the other two types reflect the absence of local kin. The Wenger network has been used in studies in Britain and Ireland (Treacy et al., 2005). However, whilst it does demonstrate some predictive value, the variables that constitute the typology are very culturally and temporally specific and the index lacks national normative data with which to compare our study (see Chapter 5). Other researchers have also sought to enumerate and classify the social networks of older people. For example, Litwin has developed a six-fold typology of social networks defined as follows: diverse, friend focused, neighbour focused, family focused, community-clan and restricted (Litwin, 2001, 2003, 2006; Litwin and Shiovitz-Ezra, 2006) and used this as a basis to predict a variety of health outcomes.

The more recent research by Phillipson and colleagues (2001b) serves to further emphasise the dominance of family-based and centred networks in the lives of older people. Indeed they argue that it is the immediate family (spouse, children, siblings) who play the largest role in the lives of older people, although the wider social network and context should not be neglected. Phillipson et al. (2001b) identify four network types based upon their composition: immediate family (60 per cent), other kin (16 per cent), non-kin (24 per cent) and care-related (1 per cent) rather than proximity, which was central to the Wenger typology. Similarly, the Lubben network scale is also dominated by kin and friendship-based measures (Lubben et al., 2006).

The pre-eminence of kinship ties in the social networks of older people provides a striking continuity with the studies of Townsend, which were dominated by kin-based relationships. As such these studies offer a strong riposte to the pessimistic social commentators who argue both for the demise of the family per se and its role in the lives of older people. However, there are a minority of the current generation of elders, six per cent overall, (eight per cent of women and three per cent of men) who have no children or siblings. A further three per cent of elders have never married, had no children and no siblings. Whilst this is very much a minority of older people it does represent a potentially vulnerable group, although as old age represents a continuation of a pre-existing lifestyle this vulnerability may be more perceived than actual, especially as friendships and wider patterns of social engagement may be 'substituted' for family networks. We must avoid the easy assumption that lack of 'blood' family means lack of social engagement or the availability of a functional social network or avenues of social support. As Phillipson's study reveals, almost a quarter of older people describe 'non-kin based' social networks. We must not forget the importance of friends and friendship in the lives of older (and younger) people (Jerrome, 1981, 1984; Phillipson et al., 1998; Jerrome and Wenger, 1999). We may speculate that, for future generations of elders, current trends in terms of marriage and family formation may increase the reliance upon non-kin based relationships for both networks and supportive linkages. This illustrates the dynamic nature of social relationships and reminds us that ageing takes place within a dynamic social context.

## Participation and activity

There is also a strong empirically based quantitative research tradition in Britain concerned with recording the patterns of social contact with family, friends and neighbours and participation in a range of 'organised' activities illustrated by older people. Such research has formed the underpinning of the social network approaches noted earlier but has also come to be seen as important in its own right. This tradition is illustrated at a national level by Hunt (1978) in her survey of older people living at home in Britain. In her study she was concerned, amongst other things, to establish the frequency of contact between older people and their family, friends and neighbours as well as their participation in a range of social activities. Similarly, a number of locally based studies such as those in South Wales (Jones et al., 1985), Clackmanan in Scotland (Bond and Carstairs, 1982) and the more recent English Longitudinal Study of Ageing (ELSA) (Barnes et al., 2006) have also carefully documented these parameters, many of which have also become incorporated into routine national social surveys such as the General Household Survey (GHS).

Within this broad tradition of enumerating social activity there are variations of emphasis and nuance between studies and they also reflect changes in the nature of social participation and engagement across society more broadly. In the case of Hunt, the location of family-based contacts was deemed important and she distinguished between visits made to family or friends and visits received from them. Recent studies undertaken as part of the General Household Survey group have not differentiated the place in which contacts take place being content to enumerate the fact that there has been contact. Typically such studies record the frequency of contact with family, friends and neighbours and participation in various activities within specific temporal reference points such as daily, weekly, in the last month and less often.

Within this tradition of research the focus is upon older people's participation – for example, do they see family members weekly, or visit the library every fortnight? There is little attention given to the nature of these engagements and the quality of the interaction or the meaning attached to it by the participants. Examination of the types of questions used by previous researchers illustrates how research has adapted and evolved in response to social change. Questions about contact with family, friends and neighbours are consistently included in studies from Townsend (1957) to the 1998 General Household Survey (Bridgwood, 2000). This reveals the not unreasonable implicit assumptions of researchers as to the high value attached to these differing contacts. Initially such questions related only to direct contacts. However, the way in which social contact takes place between family members and friends has changed markedly. Social contact can be achieved by other methods such as telephone calls, letters or now, increasingly, via electronic means and these developments are reflected in the questions asked. Townsend and Tunstall confined themselves to direct contacts; Hunt introduced notions of contact by letter and phone; and our study included email and computer-based methods of social engagement (text messaging was only just emerging at the time of our survey). Thus geographical separation does not necessarily imply neglect or lack of contact between the older person and the family. This increase in the ways that social contacts can take place means that we need to reconsider some of the simple assumptions underlying much research, which presumes that 'direct' face-to-face contacts are the most favoured and highly rated form of social contact. Furthermore, whilst this assumption may be justified for current cohorts, it may not hold true for future generations brought up on telephones, mobiles, text messaging and email and other newly emerging forms of electronic communication. The questions used by researchers have developed to include these increasingly diverse range of contacts.

We can also see that researchers give primacy to contacts with family and friends because contemporary studies ask in more detail about the nature of contacts. However, contacts with neighbours, which may be important in terms of embedding individuals within a particular spatial location, are usually researched in much less depth. For example, the General Household Survey (and our study) only ask about the frequency of contact but not the form that contact took. Indeed, as we demonstrate in Chapter 3, the status and definition of neighbours within older people's social worlds is far more complex than the straightforward, unproblematic and precise questions and phrases used by social survey researchers.

Similarly, the questions asked about participation in particular activities reflect contemporary patterns and ideas about the 'proper' spheres within which elders are expected to engage and ideas about leisure and participation more broadly. Critical evaluation of the content of long-running surveys such as the General Household Survey or Family Expenditure Survey (FES) can illustrate social change and how British society has moved from post-war austerity to a postmodern consumption-based culture. We can see this development in the questions about social participation derived from three surveys: Hunt (1978); Bond and Carstairs (1982); and Shanas et al. (1968). For example, in the survey of Clackmannan, Bond and Carstairs (1982) focused very much upon formal membership of organisations such as clubs, although only the ubiquitous 'old people's club' was specific to older people. Visits to the pub, church membership and visits to the cinema are the only forms of cultural participation represented. Shanas et al. (1968), in their comparative study of ageing in three countries, focus upon visiting, domestic activities, clubs and churches and, apart from walking, there were no obvious leisure or cultural pursuits. Similarly, the survey of Hunt (1978) focused upon hobbies rather than activities and the kinds of hobbies and pastimes reported in her study were predominantly located within the domestic sphere – respondents reported 'passive' domestic activities such as reading, watching TV and listening to the radio as well as gardening, and other domestic-based pursuits such as cooking, needlework, indoor games and repairs and redecoration. Attending church, walking and outdoor sport, as either a participant or spectator, were the only 'external' activities apart from the membership of the organisations noted above. This supports the views of Bulov et al. (2002) that the domestic and personal sphere dominates the social world of older people.

Unlike our survey (see Chapter 3 for full details) there were no questions on meals out, visits to theatre and cinema or engagement with a wider civic social world via voting or participation in voluntary activities or local political and interest groups. Indeed, this reflects the recent emergence of a more consumption and leisure-focused society in which older people, at least to some degree, now participate (Gilleard and Higgs 2000, 2002, 2005). However, we could argue that our preoccupation with non-domestic external social activities fails adequately to capture the social world of older people, which may be more locally and domestically focused than other groups within the population. Again, however, these types of questions often focus upon the presence or absence and sometimes frequency of a specific type of social activity or engagement. However, it is not just the extent of participation that is important but the value that social actors ascribe to the relationship and activity. Few studies attempt to determine this aspect of the engagement within the broader context. We know little about how participants value going to the library or attending church. Additionally, we know even less about those who do not attend such activities. For example, did those who do not participate attend such activities previously. If so why have they stopped engaging or have they never engaged in such activities?

## Loneliness, social isolation and social exclusion

Researchers, from Sheldon (1948) onwards, have shown interest in two 'pathological' extreme aspects of social relationships: loneliness and social isolation. These are often now linked under the generic term of 'social exclusion' along with other related activities such as civic engagement, access to basic services, material resources and consumption and the types of cultural and social participation noted earlier. This emphasis in research and policy, in particular upon isolation and loneliness, reflects the 'popular' stereotype that old age is a time of life which renders people especially vulnerable to such problems and, perhaps, reflects a preoccupation with the negative and problematic aspects of ageing and later life. The changed roles experienced with ageing, from employed to retired, from provider to dependant, or from spouse to widow it is argued, render older people particularly prone to these negative experiences. One key dimension of our research has been to look at how the social world of older people has changed over the past 50 years and one important dimension of this was to focus upon evaluating the prevalence of loneliness and isolation amongst specific cohorts of older people. As understanding loneliness and isolation in later life are the focus of this book, these concepts are examined in more depth in Chapter 2. Here we introduce the central themes of these concepts and develop our analysis in the next chapter. Our interest in these two topics does not, however, mean that we accept the negative stereotypes associated with old age. Whilst we must acknowledge the work undertaken in this area, as it has mapped out so much of our knowledge of social relationships in later life, we are equally if not more interested in establishing who isn't lonely or who is not isolated and what the factors are that apparently 'protect' many older people from these negative experiences.

Loneliness as a concept is theoretically, conceptually and methodologically complex (see de Jong-Gierveld, 1998; Victor et al. 2000; Jones and Hebb, 2003) but is one that has consistently attracted the attention of researchers and social commentators alike (Gibson, 2001; Seebrooke, 1973). At the most straightforward level loneliness is concerned with how individuals evaluate their overall level of social interaction. Loneliness describes the state in which there is a deficit between the individual's actual and desired level of social engagement and is distinct from being alone (time spent alone), living alone (simply a description of the household arrangements) and social isolation (which refers to the level of integration of individuals and groups into the wider social environment). It is not unusual to see these terms used interchangeably and, whilst there is undoubtedly some overlap, the degree of fit is one of the issues that we wished to explore in our study. Social isolation is portrayed as a more quantitative, empirical measurement of social engagement. This ranges from the simple tallying of social contacts in a given reference time frame, such as a week, to more sophisticated conceptualisations incorporating contacts and spatial proximity. The researcher then decides at which point along the distribution of social contacts constitutes 'isolation'. Hence a line is being drawn along a continuum to differentiate the 'isolated' from the 'non-isolated' in the same way that other continuous variables are dichotomised, such as the 'poverty' line or 'case definition thresholds' for conditions such as dementia or depression.

## Perspectives upon social relationships

There are at least four perspectives to the investigation of loneliness in later life. These were initially outlined by Townsend (1973) and developed further by Andersson (1998) and, by extension, can be applied to our understanding and analysis of social relationships in later life. The most common approach is the examination of 'peer group' patterns of relationships. This concentrates on describing the prevalence and distribution of social relationships, as measured by individual dimensions such as loneliness, isolation or social networks, amongst older people (but this perspective could, of course, be applied to other age groups) usually at a specific point in time, although a longitudinal element could be developed. Often this approach is extended as researchers seek to identify 'vulnerable' or 'at risk' groups who demonstrate one of these 'pathological' engagement states with a view to the development of screening tools to identify vulnerable elders and the development of social interventions to alleviate these states (see Lubben et al., 2006, for an example of the development of a screening tool). This approach has strong links with the 'social epidemiology' tradition towards research that we discuss further in Chapter 2 and is motivated largely by a humanitarian tradition: a desire to identify specific problems, determine the groups most at risk, develop tools to identify such people and develop interventions to alleviate the problem. 'Peer group' studies of relationships dominate the research literature, especially for older people and later life. Hence much of our knowledge base concerning the social world of older people offers a very static perspective upon what may be a very fluid and dynamic concept. The longitudinal perspective remains underdeveloped. The focus upon 'peer group' studies also results in less emphasis being placed upon locating the current pattern of relationships within a life-course perspective. How different are the observed patterns of relationships and engagement from previous phases of life?

The emphasis and focus in 'age-related' studies is to compare and contrast the experience of, for example, loneliness in later life with that experienced at other phases of the life cycle. Given the importance now attached in gerontology to understanding and articulating the life course and biographical roots to our understanding of old age and later life this is a major deficit in our evidence base. There are very few British studies that examine social relationships longitudinally and which map the ebb and flow of relationships and participation across the life course, although there are more examples from other countries such as the Manitoba Longitudinal Study of Ageing or the Survey of Health and Ageing In Europe.[1]

The other two perspectives that could be used to examine the social

---

[1] See http://www.nia.nih.gov/ResearchInformation/ScientificResources/LongitudinalStudies AllCurrent.htm for a list of all current international longitudinal studies of ageing.

relationships of older people are much less well established. Generation contrasted studies draw direct comparisons of the experience of loneliness between people of different ages. For example, we can enumerate the extent of loneliness amongst young, mid-life and older people and draw comparisons between them. Again, there are few explicit examples of such approaches as social relationships are generally perceived to be a 'problem' of old age rather than other phases of life. However, there are studies of loneliness in specific age groups such as adolescents or students and social groups such as new mothers. In the absence of general population studies asking the same question at the same time to respondents of different ages we have to use published research to attempt to make comparisons across the different age groups.

The final approach is that of preceding cohort studies which attempt to compare patterns of loneliness and social engagement amongst current cohorts of older people with those demonstrated by preceding generations of elders. As such this enables us to map out and enumerate the continuities and the changes in the social components in later life (Victor et al 2002: 2005). This, of course, requires the availability of previous studies with which to draw comparisons and a sufficiently similar methodological approach for a meaningful comparison to be made but can offer insights into the continuities and discontinuities of 'old age'.

## The study background

There is a considerable interest from researchers, policy makers and practitioners in defining, measuring and, by inference, developing interventions to promote quality of life in 'old age'. We see evidence of this in the recent report from the Deputy Prime Minister's Office (2006). Bowling (2005) provides a very comprehensive overview of this topic and illustrates how social relationships and well-being are often reduced to one domain of this concept competing for prominence with dimensions such as physical health, mental health and financial well-being. With the exception of the recent work by Phillipson and colleagues (2001b) and Treacy et al. (2005), there are few recent studies that have focused exclusively upon social relationships in later life. The

British literature concerning social relationships is dominated by the works of Townsend, Tunstall and Wenger and the community studies noted earlier. Hence this study was timely because of the lack of contemporary evidence and understanding concerning older people's social worlds.

In the 50 years since Townsend's study much has changed in the fabric of contemporary society and older people have not been immune from social change. There have been fundamental changes in the size of families and the types of households in which people live as well as other profound demographic and social changes ranging from the availability of divorce, the growth of minority population groups to increasing levels of affluence and the availability of mass consumer goods. In particular, household changes are important because they provide a context which frames much of the social world of older people. Such changes have been reported in detail elsewhere (Vincent et al., 2006; Bond et al., 2007; Johnson et al., 2005) and so we need only summarise the key changes as these form a context and rationale for our study.

The most obvious change for older people between contemporary Britain and the surveys undertaken by Townsend and Sheldon is in the nature of the households in which they live. Sheldon (1948) reported in his study of Wolverhampton that 51 per cent of older people lived with their children or grandchildren and that this was the normative pattern of social organisation. Similarly, Townsend (1957) in Bethnal Green reported that 41 per cent of women aged 60 or over and men aged 65 or over lived in two-plus generation families. These are, of course, locally based studies and we should be cautious in generalising from these specific geographical locations to the wider population. Furthermore, it is unclear if such household arrangements were arrived at by choice or reflected problems of the quantity and affordability of housing. Given a 'free choice' would families have opted to co-reside? Given this caveat both locally and nationally, the multi-generational form of living arrangement has declined markedly in the post-1945 period. Recent General Household Survey data suggest that, at most, 10 per cent of people aged 65 or over live in multi-generation households and this percentage has halved over the past 20 years and may now be as low as two per cent (Bridgewood 2000). This national change is reflected in the recent resurveys of Wolverhampton and Bethnal Green

(Phillipson et al. 1998; 2001), hence co-residence across the generations is becoming an increasingly unusual feature of Western society (Tomassini et al., 2004). Whilst there are many opinions on the desirability of this trend there is little research.

The converse of the decrease of the multi-generational household has been the development of single-person households. In 1901 it is estimated that only five per cent of households consisted of single persons (Thane, 2000). This had increased to 11 per cent in 1961, 17 per cent in 1971 and 31 per cent in 2005 (2006). This trend towards solo living is not unique to older people. Indeed one of the most pervasive trends over the past 50 years has been the increase in solo living across the generations. The percentage of households consisting of a single person of pension age has increased little since 1971 from 12 per cent to 15 per cent in 2005 (Fido et al., 2006). Over the same period single-person households consisting of a person under pension age increased from five per cent to 16 per cent (2006). In 1961 64 per cent of single-person households were 'pensioners'; by 2005 this had decreased to 48 per cent (2006). In pre-industrial England probably less than 10 per cent of the older population lived alone and this was probably stable until the 1950s (Thane, 2000).

Even given the caveat that reliance upon local surveys in areas of acute housing problems such as east London may overstate the extent of social change, it is evident that in the space of 50 years there has been a fundamental and profound change in the living arrangements of older people (and by extension other age groups as well). These changes are not unique to Great Britain but are observable in other developed countries (United Nations, 2005). However, these data simply state changes in the pattern of household organisation. We cannot presume that because older people do not now live in multi-generational households that they are not members of multi-genera-tional family groups. We, again, cannot use such data to infer that older people are not part of multi-generational families. Grundy and Shelton (2001) and Shelton and Grundy (2000) report that 75 per cent of those aged 60 and over are part of families which include three or more generations. Indeed, given greater life expectancy, it is usual for families to consist of four or five generations. People can be both grandparents and grandchildren simultaneously! Although there has been a spatial separation of families into separate living groups, family ties are clearly being maintained and older people, like most of the rest of the population, consider themselves to be members of wider family groups. Again, declines in co-residence cannot be used to make any inferences about the nature and quality of relationships between family members. Similarly, we need to develop an analysis of family relationships which is more sophisticated than a simple 'proximity equals quality and intimacy' and 'distance militates against intimacy and support' axiom.

There is an extensive body of work linking 'living alone' with a variety of negative physical and mental health outcomes including anxiety, depression, cognitive decline and psychological distress (see van Gelder et al., 2006). However, closer analysis of the research indicates that those who live alone are not a homogeneous group. There are qualitative differences in health outcomes, especially in terms of emotional health between men and women. However, researchers rarely distinguish between those for whom living alone is an established pattern from those for whom living alone is both a recent event and often a traumatic one resultant from bereavement. Hence this is another element of the social world of older people that merits further and closer analysis.

In our focus upon the growth of single-person households and the corresponding decline in multi-generational households we have failed to remark on the third and equally important component of the changing household arrangements of older people: the increase in the number of married or cohabiting couples maintaining independent households from children, siblings or other relatives. In the survey by Sheldon (1948) only 16 per cent of all respondents lived as a married couple alone and of those who were married only 35 per cent lived solely with their spouse. In contrast, in 2001 47 per cent of those aged 65 years or over lived solely with their spouse and, of those who were married, 91 per cent live with their spouse alone. The decline in multi-generational households has not simply resulted in the increase in older people living alone but also in a rise of older couples living independently from their children or siblings (or both). This change reflects a number of inter-related trends including the establishment of independent households by children at an earlier age, often before marriage, the establishment of long-term relationships, and greater longevity for both men and women. A much less noted trend is that, because of the well observed reductions in mortality for both men and women, couples who marry or cohabit can expect to 'grow old together' and to live together in their own home in old age. Whilst less remarked than the percentages of older people living alone or the decrease in multi-generational households, both of which can be indirectly presented as evidence of our less caring and neglectful treatment of older people, the increase in percentage of older couples living independently in later life has had an equally profound influence upon the experience of later life and in framing the context within which old age is experienced.

These changes are summarised in Chapter 3 (Table 3.1) which compares the characteristics of our current study population with those reported by key studies of Sheldon, Townsend and others. It is easy to overlook the magnitude of these demographic changes and to underestimate how much the change in such variables has influenced the experience of old age and later life. Of course when attempting to examine changes in social relationships across different cohorts of older people these trends will exert a key if unquantifiable influence.

The project upon which this book is largely based was conducted in order to address a number of limitations of previous research concerning our understanding of the experience of social relationships in later life. We sought to undertake a contemporary study that would address the major limitations in our knowledge base and the changing social landscape within which older people play out their social relationships. In particular, our study sought to respond to the following imitations:

◆ Family and household change. As noted earlier there has been significant social change in the past 50 years, not least in terms of living arrangements, family and friendship networks, which may have had an impact upon social participation and social exclusion, especially social isolation and loneliness.

◆ Dominance of local perspective. Recent studies have been conducted in specific geographical areas (e.g. North Wales and east London). These studies are highly informative. However, they may lack generalisability because of the specific localities studied. For example, Wenger's work in North Wales is focused upon a specific type of rural community within a specific Welsh-speaking context. The transferability of the findings of studies from specific contexts needs to be established via the generation of nationally representative data.

◆ Conceptual confusion. Studies of social engagement and exclusion have rarely clearly distinguished between concepts such as networks, social support or isolation and loneliness. Relationships have been presumed with factors such as living alone with little empirical evidence of the actual degree of overlap. Furthermore, traditional survey methods may have perpetuated the public account (Cornwell, 1984) of isolation and loneliness with older people (or indeed other age groups) being unwilling to report the presence of such potentially stigmatising experiences. Little attempt has been made to investigate the value and meaning of the concepts to older people themselves. Measures of isolation that focus on direct contact with family members may be inappropriate and underestimate the importance of indirect contact (e.g. telephone, email) to older people. We have presumed that quantity and quality of contacts are linked. This may not be the case.

◆ Adopting a life-course perspective. Our evidence base is dominated by peer group, cross-sectional studies of social engagement. We have failed to adopt a 'life-course' perspective by distinguishing between those who have always been social isolates (or lonely) from those who recently became isolated (or lonely). In policy terms these are two distinct groups and research has not explored the theoretical possibility that in later life people might become less isolated or lonely.

◆ Predictors and explanations for isolation and loneliness are relatively poorly investigated in earlier British studies and the North American experience may not be generalisable to the UK. The lack of appropriate statistical tools may in the past have militated against the sophisticated modelling of factors predicting isolation and loneliness, which is now feasible. For example, research has consistently linked living alone with decreased social participation and increased levels of loneliness and isolation. However, from our basic social epidemiology of old age we know that those who live alone are more likely to be older, female and suffering from chronic physical or mental health problems. How much of the link between living alone and exclusion is, in fact, the result of, for example, poor health rather than living alone? Multivariate statistical techniques enable us to explore the complexity of these linkages and identify a set of 'risk factors' and also explore the potential identification of factors that 'protect' against social exclusion.

More specifically the aims of our study were to contribute to the theoretical and empirical understanding of later life by examining the extent and meaning of isolation and loneliness in later life to the individual and by examining the relationship between loneliness, social isolation and living alone and to contribute to policy and practice by identifying factors protective against isolation and loneliness.

The specific objectives of our project were:

- To describe the prevalence of social isolation and loneliness amongst older people living in the community, by the collection of survey data and 'depth' interviews.

- To contribute to our understanding of secular trends in the experience of quality of life amongst older people by comparing our results with the classic community studies of Sheldon, Townsend and Tunstall.

- To contribute to knowledge and understanding of later life by investigating the relationship between loneliness and social isolation and living alone for older people.

- To contribute to policy and practice by identifying the factors, resources and coping mechanisms that protect older people from experiencing loneliness and isolation.

In this chapter we have outlined the key concepts and issues that we will be addressing within our book and indicated the structure of our argument. In subsequent chapters we consider in more detail the parameters of the social world of older people, describe our study methods and characterise the people who participated in the study and provide a comprehensive perspective upon the social environment and world inhabited by older people in contemporary society.

# 2

# Loneliness and social isolation:

## Issues of theory and method

In gerontology the concepts of 'loneliness' and 'social isolation' have often been used to characterise the social world of older people and as an indicator of their quality of life. Like many other social science concepts they are taken-for-granted ideas from everyday life. It is often contended that loneliness and social isolation are common problems of later life that lead to widespread unhappiness and social exclusion. In Chapter 1 we highlighted how a dominant tradition in gerontology focused on the problems of later life as a response to the humanistic concerns and the general push for social improvement that emerged during the reconstruction of the post-war era. We argued that loneliness and social isolation have become 'pathological' concepts that focus on the negative aspects of social relations at the expense of understanding the positive side of later life. This problem-oriented approach dominated gerontology for many decades and the tradition has been characterised as empirical and atheoretical. Gerontology and the study of ageing have been described as 'data rich and theory poor' (Birren and Bengston, 1988: 74). One consequence has been that concepts like loneliness and social isolation have been widely used but rarely contested since their emergence in the social and behavioural science writings of the 1950s. Yet, despite their self-evident meaning both concepts remain conceptually and theoretically problematic.

In this chapter we provide an account of the use of loneliness and social isolation in gerontological theory and will contest the dominant paradigm that problematises, stigmatises and medicalises the social position of older people in post-modernity. We will use our interest in the social relationships in later life to make broader theoretical points about the subject area and the state of gerontological theory, knowledge and research activity. Many of the early theories in gerontology such as disengagement theory (Cumming and Henry, 1961) and activity theory (Havighurst, 1963) and, more recently, the re-emergence of a theory of successful ageing (Rowe and Kahn, 1997) have been highly 'judgemental', offering moral statements, values and dictates that suggest that there is a correct way to age. By extension, these theoretical propositions indicate that there are also deviant patterns of adaptation to the very real physiological and social changes that accompany ageing. We may characterise such deviant positions as 'growing old disgracefully', rather than ageing gracefully, as is typified by the sentiments of the poem *Warning* by Jenny Joseph (Box 2.1). As we all age we experience changes in our interactions, relationships and attachments with others, yet we would argue that changes in our emotional and social experiences may not be as remarkable, prevalent or damaging as many commentators would have us believe.

We do not wish to deny the often traumatic significant emotional impact of loss and bereavement in later life or the very real social and political consequences of social exclusion for older people, either individually or collectively. Rather we wish to challenge the apocalyptical and highly negative and stereotyped views of so many politicians, policymakers and health and welfare professionals whose professional gaze overlooks the positive, rewarding and memorable experiences of later life or the way that older people can adapt and grow in response to the physical, social and psychological challenges that often accompany ageing. We suggest that the focus upon the negative and pathological aspects of social relationships leads to the neglect of the 'normal' and non-problematic aspects of older people's lives and the ways that they respond to social challenges. Our empirical data attempt to provide evidence about the 'normal', to contextualise the 'pathological' and to look for the historical and biographical framework within which social relationships are enacted.

Before presenting our empirical evidence this chapter focuses upon clarifying our understanding of loneliness and social isolation through a review of these concepts in theory and empirical research. To do this we will need to examine questions of ontology, theory, epistemology and method. Our purpose in critically reviewing these concepts is because of their importance in shaping our understanding of the social

---

**Box 2.1** *Warning*

When I am an old woman I shall wear purple
With a red hat which doesn't go, and doesn't suit me.
And I shall spend my pension on brandy and summer gloves
And satin sandals, and say we've no money for butter.
I shall sit down on the pavement when I'm tired
And gobble up samples in shops and press alarm bells
And run my stick along the public railings
And make up for the sobriety of my youth.
I shall go out in my slippers in the rain
And pick the flowers in other people's gardens
And learn to spit.

You can wear terrible shirts and grow more fat
And eat three pounds of sausages at a go
Or only bread and pickle for a week
And hoard pens and pencils and beermats and things in boxes.

But now we must have clothes that keep us dry
And pay our rent and not swear in the street
And set a good example for the children.
We must have friends to dinner and read the papers.

But maybe I ought to practise a little now?
So people who know me are not too shocked and surprised
When suddenly I am old, and start to wear purple

Jenny Joseph

*Source:* Martz, S. (ed.) (1987) When I am an Old Woman I Shall Wear Purple. Papier-Mache Press, Watsonville, Ca., p. 1.

---

relationships of older people and also as a means of illustrating the narrowness of the gaze which researchers have cast upon this topic. We suggest that this observation may apply more widely to topics such as health and illness or 'unmet' need. Our focus upon these two key issues does not mean that we accept the partial view that they suggest. Rather we are using these concepts to illustrate many of the key issues underpinning contemporary social gerontological research and as a way of focusing our topic of interest. The study of loneliness and isolation (and the non-lonely and non-isolated) contributes to our understanding of social relationships in later life in a much more generic way than simply concentrating upon a single type of relationship (marriage or friendship) or activity (attending church or participating in an exercise class) can.

## Loneliness and social isolation in gerontological research

The emergence of loneliness and social isolation as social and behavioural science concepts can be traced back through the founding writings of the two major disciplines which underpin social gerontology, most notably sociology and psychology. Marx's concept of alienation (Bottomore and Rubel, 1965) and Durkheim's concept of *anomie* (Durkheim, 1952) in sociology and ideas about the self (Cooley, 1902; Holstein and Gubrium, 2000; Mead, 1934) in sociology and social psychology offer a useful starting point for our theoretical thinking in this area. However, it was in the British community surveys of older people in the 1940s and 1950s that loneliness and social isolation amongst the older population emerged as contemporary social issues about which social commentators, politicians and policymakers could all agree that 'something should be done' (Thane, 2000). Here the focus is upon the emergence of loneliness and isolation as empirical concepts rather than as theoretical concepts. The Institute of Community Studies in the East End of London (Briggs, 2001) was at the vanguard of this tradition, as is evident from the writings of Marris (1958, 1986), Townsend (1957), Townsend and Tunstall (1968) and Tunstall (1966). Despite the methodological variability of these studies two consistent and compelling interpretations emerged: the continuing importance of family and kinship in the lives of the population in general and older people more specifically; and the exclusion (socially and materially) of a minority of those included within the compass of these investigations.

Much good work emerged from these studies and many have become 'classics' of social science. Some of these studies served to democratise social science with rich descriptions of the daily lives of ordinary citizens in differing geographical communities or settings such as Townsend's (1962) book on long-stay care, *The Last Refuge*. This timely book was one of the first to look critically at the lives of older people in environments or settings that were away from public gaze. These studies in some ways foreshadow the current interests in user involvement in research by putting 'ordinary' people and their lives at the centre of the research, although the research questions were clearly not set by the research participants, nor were they in control of the research process.

The complex and largely enduring links between families and communities were exposed to public gaze. In doing this the popular post-war myths of family breakdown resultant from the creation of the Welfare State and the lack of integration of older people within family settings were vigorously challenged. However, with regard to social relationships and the social world of older people an important paradox quickly emerged. Amongst the minority of older people who seemed objectively to be isolated or excluded there were many who reported contentment with their lives and levels of social engagement. Conversely others, often the central focus of a large family and kinship network, reported that they experienced loneliness and desolation. This paradox posed the essential ontological questions about what are the nature of the knowable and the nature of reality. How could we reconcile such apparently contradictory empirical findings? However, the emphasis of this work was in social accounting a form of twentieth-century social arithmetic rather than with issues of social theory. We have to look elsewhere for the philosophical and theoretical concepts underpinning work concerned with loneliness and isolation across the lifecourse.

## Loneliness, social isolation and individual lived experience[1]

From a philosophical perspective there are two fundamental questions for our research project and other social scientists working in this broad area. Do loneliness and social isolation exist in the 'real world'? Are these entities that we can objectively describe, define and measure empirically? Furthermore, can we describe how experiences of loneliness and social isolation vary within the older population, over time

---

[1] This section is adapted from Bond, J. and Corner, L. (2004) *Quality of Life and Older People*. Buckingham: Open University Press, pp. 101–2.

or between different societies? Are these social phenomena that we can identify, predict and ameliorate via the development of individual or group-based social interventions? Alternatively, are these inherently subjective experiences mediated and described through the gaze of a particular individual, at a particular time and within a specific socio-environmental context? Are these fundamentally personal and relativist concepts that are in no way measurable and indeed where measurement is a meaningless concept? The answers to these questions are rooted within the differing philosophical traditions that underpin social gerontological research and the social sciences more broadly and which are the bedrock of the development of knowledge.

Social scientists, who argue that loneliness and social isolation are entities that we can describe, measure objectively and 'predict', that these are 'real' experiences of the real world and therefore something that we can potentially control, may be classified as positivists. Researchers working in this tradition are predominantly concerned with establishing the extent of specific social phenomena and with describing their distribution within and between different social groups. Additionally they may also be interested in trying to 'predict' those at risk of experiencing phenomena through the development of screening procedures and interventions to combat and alleviate these states.

From a positivist perspective the paradox of the lack of fit between objective measures of loneliness and social isolation and reported experiences can be explained in two ways: measurement error and respondent error. Explanations in terms of measurement error suggest that the quality of our measures or indicators of loneliness and social isolation are poor: they are insufficiently designed to measure precisely and accurately the phenomena of interest. The lack of precision results in poor estimates of prevalence and insufficient accuracy in the identification of the affected individuals. In traditional screening terms we would have too many 'false positives', people being inaccurately labelled as 'lonely', and too many 'false negatives', lonely people being inaccurately labelled as 'not lonely'. Alternatively, the observed lack of fit between accounts of loneliness and isolation relates to the trustworthiness (or lack of it) of subjectivist accounts. In essence our 'respondents' are being untruthful or untrustworthy in their responses to our questions, perhaps because they do not wish to appear 'inadequate' to an interviewer by 'admitting' that they are lonely. The explanation for this disjuncture between differing accounts is seen as a reflection of either our imprecise or inaccurate ways of operationalising our concepts of loneliness and social isolation and a suspicion as to the veracity of 'subjective' accounts. That objective definitions may be constructed differently by different individuals or social groups is not an explanation considered valid by positivists who look for their explanation of dissonance and 'noise' in terms of issues of concept formation and measurement and, perhaps, a disinclination to 'believe' their respondents.

The failure of positivists to accept the role of individuals and groups in constructing socially based realities could appear to be rather naïve in the face of the paradox of objective and reported subjective experience of social relationships and the complexity and fluidity of the social environment. If loneliness and social isolation remain objective features of everyday life, driven by the natural world and subject to natural laws, their real natures are seen through the eyes of humans who interpret the real world and provide their own personal accounts of 'real' social phenomena. Social scientists who have adapted positivism in this way are known as post-positivists. They still retain the notion that loneliness and social isolation are objective concepts, indeed that is central to their philosophical position. However, this is linked to the recognition that objective definitions of loneliness and social isolation are constructed differently by different members of society, that such constructions are specific to particular societies and that they are temporally defined. This allows for the construction of social phenomena to vary over time, between different societies and cultures and within and between differing social groups. Hence objective social phenomena are seen as being sensitive to the social context.

This 'post-positivist' approach, which accepts that objective social phenomena can be 'socially constructed and interpreted', reflects the broad position taken by critical gerontology (Biggs 1997; Biggs et al., 2003; Holstein and Minkler, 2003; Baars et al., 2006). This coalition of ideas brings together the perspectives of feminism and post-Marxism plus new challenges such as globalisation and posits that the nature of objective reality is mediated by the values of individual actors as members of a complex, stratified and constantly changing society. These perspectives may partly explain our paradox of the disjuncture between objective experience and reported subjective experience of older people but they also suggest a new range of research questions. From this perspective the important question then becomes what values and whose values should govern the way we view experiences and entities such as loneliness and social isolation? Clearly the choice of a specific value system tends to empower and enfranchise certain individuals and groups at the expense of others and the definition of loneliness and social isolation becomes a political act and one that constructs and reconstructs the nature of the concepts. Another example of this argument may be demonstrated by the concept of 'unmet need'. Since the seminal paper by Williamson et al. (1964) numerous surveys, both local and national, have demonstrated that older people living at home experience a range of 'health problems' that are 'unknown' to the primary health care team and social services departments. Typical of such problems are hearing and sight impairments, limitations of mobility and problems with instrumental activities of daily living (e.g. cleaning and shopping). However, such surveys impose an external definition of 'need' or 'problem'. Few of these studies ask the older people themselves if the issue identified is problematic. For example, an older person may have mobility limitations resultant from arthritis and have changed their daily routine rather than seeking medical help. As such the imposition of the label 'problem' or 'unmet need' is not one which the older person would necessarily accept or recognise and the imposition of which may have more to do with the battle for resources within health services than anything else.

We challenge the objective nature of loneliness and social isolation accepted by the realist and critical realist ontologies of positivism, post-positivism and critical gerontology. Rather we view loneliness and social isolation as subjective lived experiences that exist in the form of multiple realities constructed and reconstructed by individual older people within the context of their different lives and life histories. We offer three related arguments to support our position. First, our argument takes the conventional composition of the constructionist account. If loneliness and social isolation are to have objective realities like a tree or a house then it is essential that 'scientific' facts about the nature and extent of loneliness and social isolation are collected independently of any theoretical framework used to define them. That such independence between the language of observation and theory is now recognised by philosophers of science to be impossible (Hesse, 1980) means that objective reality only exists in the context of a mental framework or construct for thinking about it. Thus objective loneliness and social isolation can only exist within theoretical frameworks that describe characteristics of loneliness and social isolation in pre-determined, uncontentious and fixed ways. It is unlikely that there exists consensus about the definitions presented.

Second, because of the philosophical problems of induction no theory can ever be fully tested, although we may get close to this 'gold standard' for some phenomena. Whilst we are unable to say with complete certainty 'that the sun will always rise in the east', our astronomical theories, observations and predictions are reasonably robust on the 'truth' or certainty of this prediction. However, unlike some physical or natural phenomena, there will always be a number of competing and plausible theories to explain social phenomena such as loneliness and social isolation. As we shall see in a later section, explanations for loneliness can be found in the writings of theoreticians from a variety of differing perspectives and we would argue that no unequivocal explanations of such complex social phenomena are likely to ever be possible. There will continue to be many constructions and objective reality will therefore only be seen within the context of a given theoretical framework and through the gaze of individual theorists and researchers, which will vary in response to changes and developments in theoretical frameworks for understanding social life. Such a conclusion has implications for how we approach the empirical study of these phenomena.

Third, we acknowledge that studying loneliness and social isolation is not a value-free activity and that facts are, to a lesser or greater degree, value laden. So not only are loneliness and social isolation seen through the gaze of individual theorists but also through that of specific social values multiplying the constructions available. Again these values are subject to modification and change. Thus ontologically there are always many interpretations of what is meant by loneliness and social isolation and there exists no scientific or unequivocal process for establishing the ultimate objective reality of these aspects of social life, as is the case for other social phenomena such as social exclusion or social capital.

Rather we propose that there is no viable alternative to relativism and the idea of multiple realities when thinking about loneliness and social isolation, irrespective of the population. The meaning of loneliness and social isolation lives in the individual's mind and seeking their specific and personal accounts may be the only way to access them. Hence rather than trying to determine the inalienable 'truth' about social relationships our research embraces the pluralism implicit within the task of understanding the social world of specific groups of social actors, in our case older people. As such we therefore use a variety of methodological approaches to capture these multiple realities. We do not seek to present a simple 'answer' to the question: What is the extent of loneliness and isolation amongst older people in contemporary Britain? Rather we seek to convey the complexity of the varying research perspectives of the differing ways of answering these questions and present the complex and competing accounts that emerge as a way of illustrating the depth and complexity that characterises the social lives of older people.

## Constructions of loneliness and social isolation

Since the early work of Sheldon (1948) and Townsend (1957) various constructions of loneliness and social isolation have emerged which, in part, help to explain the conceptual confusion around these everyday 'common-sense' ideas. By examining some of the key works in this area we can expose the variable nature of the concepts captured by the apparently constant and consistent terms loneliness and isolation. This review is not intended to be comprehensive. Rather it is focused upon the exemplars and influential writers who serve as illustrations of the wider points we wish to raise.

One important contributory factor to this conceptual confusion derives from the often made suggestion that loneliness and isolation reflect the objective and subjective side of the same concept; namely a deficit of social interactions. Townsend (Townsend and Tunstall, 1968) describes loneliness as a subjective experience resulting from an absence or loss of social interactions and social isolation as an objective enumeration of social interaction. At least in principle Townsend argued that the level of social interaction for an individual can be both unambiguously quantified and an arbitrary line drawn below which individuals could be categorised as 'isolated'. The analogy here is with the way we assess income levels and establish an amount which determines 'the poverty line'. Hence isolation was seen as both quantifiable and categorisable in a way in which we could define other 'pathological' or 'deviant states'; we could draw an unambiguous line separating the engaged from the isolated and the included from the excluded.

This distinction between the two states of loneliness and isolation is, however, problematic. It implies that loneliness and social isolation are at least in part the same social phenomenon and, because it says nothing about the quality of those interactions, it is merely quantity that matters and all interactions are attributed the same statistical weight or 'social value'. We feel that it is both naïve and simplistic to presume such an unsophisticated 'equal value' rating of social interactions and to presume that more is inherently better. For this reason we see social isolation, like loneliness, as a subjective experience and a social experience that is distinctive although sharing many common characteristics with the experience of loneliness. This shared view suggests that social isolation means the universal and necessary lack of communion between individuals (Townsend and Tunstall, 1968) and a detachment from the socio-spatial context of daily life.

We must distinguish between the notion of 'isolation' or 'aloneness' defined either by spatial or temporal separation from others and 'social isolation'. We all experience aloneness in our everyday lives since, with few exceptions, we all experience aspects of our lives alone. We may work on our own or partake of recreational activities such as running or walking on our own or we may live on our own rather than in a larger household. It is easy to assume a direct link between living alone and isolation and loneliness. Therefore, assumptions about the nature and quality of individuals' social relationships are made simply from a description of their living arrangements. Whilst there is an overlap between notions of aloneness, living alone, social isolation and loneliness these concepts do not demonstrate perfect symmetry and we need to examine the complexity of these states individually and the relationships between them

The conceptual confusion that abounds in this specific area of research is extended by the use of different terminology within the loneliness research community, although terminological inexactitude is not the exclusive preserve of researchers in this area. In particular, given the influence of his writings on the subject of loneliness, we should highlight the conceptual distinction made by Weiss (1973) between emotional loneliness, defined as an 'affective state' produced by the absence of an attachment figure, and social loneliness or the absence of an accessible social network or recognised social roles. At a broad conceptual level these two terms approximately equate to the definitions of 'loneliness' and 'social isolation' articulated by Townsend and Tunstall (1968). However, for Weiss these ideas exhibit different theoretical characteristics although both subjective concepts derive from the positive or post-positivist paradigm rather than a more constructivist approach. In his more recent reflections on loneliness Weiss suggests that there is a greater complexity than this initial typology might suggest and has argued that the experience of these states may be different for older people to those of younger adults, adolescents or children. In particular, he reflects on the paradox of the very large numbers of older people who are free of loneliness even when without an obvious attachment figure. He also suggests that for older people social loneliness may have greater significance given that older people 'seem to display a new appreciation for kin' (Weiss, 1987: 14) and, perhaps, by extension for friends and neighbours and other forms of social participation and engagement. The conceptual distinction between emotional and social is one that has underpinned the development of a variety of different measures and remains important for contemporary social surveys of older people. We shall return to this issue later in this chapter when we consider measures of loneliness.

During the 1970s the study of loneliness and social isolation in old age became a fashionable and fruitful research topic for gerontologists both in Britain and North America. This research concern crossed the disciplinary divide and included sociologists, psychologists and those concerned with social policy. Although various definitions of loneliness have been suggested by different scholars and researchers from within different disciplinary perspectives, such as psychology and sociology, there was agreement about the broad concept of loneliness at the time. Three essential key characteristics of loneliness were distilled from a review of the definitions and concepts (Peplau and Perlman, 1982: 3):

- Loneliness results from the deficiencies in a person's social relationships.

- Loneliness is a subjective experience.

- The experience of loneliness is unpleasant and distressing.

This consensus view of the key attributes of the concept of loneliness is exemplified by de Jong-Gierveld in her review (de Jong-Gierveld, 1998: 73–4) in which she presents her own definition of the concept as:

> Loneliness is a situation experienced by the individual as one where there is an unpleasant or inadmissible lack of (quality of) certain relationships. This includes situations in which the number of existing relationships is smaller than is considered desirable or admissible, as well as situations where the intimacy one wishes for has not been realized. Thus loneliness is seen to involve the manner in which the person perceives, experiences, and evaluates his or her isolation and lack of communication with other people.

Whilst we can trace the development of a broad consensus concerning the 'key attributes' of the notion of loneliness, social isolation is both more problematic and elusive. To the best of our knowledge there does not seem to have been a parallel consensus to emerge. The construction of the concept of social isolation has not been so well reviewed perhaps because the definition of the 'precise' level of engagement that defined isolation, the specification of a 'case-definition threshold', offered more potential for disputes between researchers than for establishing consensus. To some degree the concern with isolation and its definition and identification has been absorbed within the social networks research perspective (Lubben et al., 2006) and more recently the social exclusion research agenda (Scharf et al., 2005b and 2005c; Scharf, 2005).

The assumptions and values of positivism and post-positivism clearly emerge from this brief summary of loneliness and isolation. By conceptualising loneliness, and by implication social isolation, as a deficiency in a person's social relationships the perspective problematises and individualises loneliness and pathologises the individual's social relationships. This leads to the 'blaming' of individuals for their situation and the development of a type of 'personal-tragedy' theory of ageing which has been very well argued and articulated in the disability studies literature (Oliver, 1990). Such an approach does not encourage looking at the wider social context within which the older person is located. Rather the focus and analysis or understanding is located at the individual level. We would certainly not challenge the idea that both loneliness and social isolation, as we all understand them in everyday life, are unpleasant and distressing experiences. We do, however, strongly challenge the view that it is the individual who is lonely or socially isolated who is to blame and that the broader social context within which older people are located is immaterial.

## Issues of theory in researching loneliness and social isolation

In general, theoretical questions are concerned with how we explain past events and predict, or attempt to predict, future events, although this is contingent upon the perspective adopted. Positivists, post-positivists and critical theorists often invoke theory in prediction. Constructionists use theory as a means of explaining or understanding the past; they are much less concerned with prediction. This may be because there is less concern with identifying those 'at risk' and sub-sequently intervening and 'curing' the identified problem.

A range of behavioural and social science disciplines have developed theories about loneliness and social isolation (Perlman and Peplau, 1982; Marangoni and Ickes, 1989). Reviews of these theories add to the confusion around both concepts, rather than offering clarification because of the use of differing taxonomies of theories and linguistic variation. However, providing an overview of the key theories helps toward an understanding of the diversity of concepts discussed in the literature. Again our focus here is upon highlighting the key positions in the debates rather than a comprehensive review.

### Psychodynamic, personality and behavioural perspectives

Many of the early ideas about loneliness were generated from within a broadly Freudian psychodynamic tradition. The development of psychodynamic theory stems largely from clinical observations of individuals with various pathologies that differentiate them from 'normal' individuals. Indeed, perspectives deriving from clinical observations and the study of individuals or groups with defined pathologies have been highly influential in the development of gerontological theory, research and practice more generally. The use of clinical observations and populations to develop theories about and make empirical observations about 'normal ageing' is both problematic and contentious. As an example we can cite the studies based upon populations receiving services who demonstrate a profile that is distinct from the rest of the population.

Loneliness (as opposed to being alone or lonesome) viewed from this essentially Freudian perspective is characterised as abnormal. It is defined as a deviant state demonstrated in those who are clearly outwith the norm. We suggest that the psychodynamic characterisation of loneliness as pathology has contributed to the medicalisation (Conrad and Schneider, 1980; Ballard and Elston, 2005) and stigmatisation (Goffman, 1968) of this dimension of human experience. Psychodynamic theory seeks explanations of loneliness, at any age, which are located in childhood including poor parent–child interactions, premature weaning and other experiences of infancy. The focus of the Freudian tradition maps how factors within the individual such as traits and intra-psychic conflicts lead to loneliness. The importance of this early tradition in pathologising and medicalising loneliness should not be underestimated as the continued interest in the links (or otherwise) between loneliness and depression demonstrate and the argument that loneliness is 'merely' sub-clinical depression and not a distinct entity attests (Barg et al., 2006; Cacioppo et al., 2006). From a social constructionist perspective this is a highly inadequate account of loneliness, taking little account of the social context in which individuals live or of their own interpretation of loneliness and is an explanation offered at the level of the individual. Furthermore, the explanatory framework, with its roots in early infant experiences, is both 'deterministic' and relegates the importance of other life experiences and other stages of the life course.

Personality theories have evolved from the psychodynamic tradition in a number of ways and in line with that tradition's use of clinical experience and observation to speculate on some of the potential causes of loneliness. An early example of this approach was the phenomenological perspective of Carl Rogers (1970). This approach should not be confused with the phenomenological philosophy of Husserl. Rogers' analysis assumes that society forces individuals to act in restricted and socially approved ways. His 'self theory' of personality suggests that the demands of the social pressures to conform leads to a discrepancy between one's true inner self and the self presented in everyday life – a phenomenological discrepancy in one's self-concept. Loneliness is experienced by these individuals when they drop their external persona to get in touch with their inner selves and, according to Rogers, the belief that their real selves are unlovable 'keeps people locked in their loneliness' (Rogers, 1970: 121). In contrast to the psychodynamic tradition, this approach puts greater emphasis on the influence of an individual's current experience and social context than childhood influences but this remains a negative perspective on a social state that does not seem to offer any positive possibilities and again is an explanatory framework that focuses upon the individual and blames the individual.

The existentialist approach has also emerged from clinical practice but is rather less commonly cited in loneliness research than other theoretical perspectives, although there are now measures that derive from this theoretical stance (Mayers and Svartberg, 2001; Mayers et al., 2002; Sand and Strang, 2006). It takes as its starting point the idea that each of us is ultimately alone since no one else can ever experience our real thoughts and feelings. As individuals we share only those inner thoughts with others that we choose to. This may represent a complete or partial sharing. Unlike the previous two approaches, for the existentialist, loneliness has a positive aspect by giving individuals the opportunity to act reflexively, to encounter themselves and potentially build an understanding of themselves. Also loneliness is not seen as a minority or deviant state but rather is part and parcel of 'normal' human experience. Thus, rather than look for causes of loneliness this approach seeks to encourage people to overcome their fear of lone-liness and to use loneliness positively (Moustakas, 1972; Moustakas and Mous, 2004). From a constructionist perspective we are sympa-thetic to the role of reflexivity in understanding loneliness. However, the approach fails to delineate between the subjectivity of loneliness and the subjectivity of being alone. Although the approach does not deny the pain of loneliness for some, it does ignore the potentially negative effects of being alone (Weiss, 1973).

Within the positivist and post-positivist paradigm, empirical studies have examined a number of personality and behavioural characteristics of people who have been defined as lonely or not lonely. For example, Marangoni and Ickes (1989) highlight positive associations with shyness, self-consciousness, depression, negative self-concept, inhibited sociability and unassertiveness. Negative associations reported include: self-esteem, social risk taking, extraversion and perceptions of own social skills. Similar associations have been reported for young people (Mahon et al., 2006). Again, however, there is a consistent failure to examine the role of the 'social context' in explaining loneliness and isolation in later life.

## Psychological perspectives

The phenomenological tradition in psychology highlights the importance of cognitive processes in understanding how individuals experience social phenomena such as loneliness or isolation. Cognition is advanced as the mediating factor between deficits in sociability or significant relationships and the experience of loneliness or isolation (Peplau et al., 1982). Two similar theoretical approaches have been used to explain loneliness in this way: attribution theory (Lunt, 1991; Peplau et al., 1982) and self-discrepancy theory (Peplau et al., 1982). From these perspectives the gap between expectations of social relationships and perceived experience is a characteristic of loneliness. An individual who by 'objective' standards would not be expected to be lonely may experience feelings of loneliness where the frequency or quality of social contacts fall below a desired level (de Jong-Gierveld and Raadschelders, 1982; Peplau and Perlman, 1982). An individual's attributional style may also reflect social skills deficits that themselves influence the maintenance and chronicity of loneliness. A review of studies supports the finding that lonely individuals tend to attribute their loneliness and interpersonal deficits to uncontrollable external causes and exhibit dysfunctional attitudes such as fear of rejection and insecurity in interpersonal relations, social embarrassment in social interactions and high levels of social anxiety (Marangoni and Ickes, 1989). Thus, in general, it would appear that both qualitative and quantitative aspects of an individual's social relations may be mediated by specific types of behaviour within interpersonal relationships as well as by cognitive processes.

47

Within psychology there have also been two approaches to loneliness that have given primary emphasis to unmet needs: social developmental and social support approaches. The social developmental approach has its historical roots in neo-Freudian psychoanalysis, highlighting the importance of social relationships in providing fulfilment of our needs for human intimacy. Earlier theorists characterised loneliness in terms of deficits in social relations, but it is probably Bowlby's work on attachment (Bowlby, 1971) that has had most influence on the social developmental approach through the proposed relationship between early attachment processes during infancy and adult loneliness. The suggestion here is that in adult life similar attachment bonds occur in intimate adult relationships as existed in childhood. Just as infant–parent patterns can be characterised as *secure, avoidant* or *anxious-ambivalent,* so too can the attachment patterns of adults in intimate relationships be so characterised. From these theoretical ideas has also emerged the importance of the intimate attachment or significant confidant in adult relationships which has had a profound influence upon studies of quality of life and social engagement (Weiss, 1973).

There is a significant body of literature evaluating the importance of intimate relationships as a defence against the vicissitudes of old age and which has investigated the presence or absence of such ties and demonstrates a preoccupation with social support. In the development of the social support approach, loneliness is conceived as the absence of a significant attachment, an absence that limits self-esteem and self-worth and which then has negative influence upon 'quality of life'. The key points to note here are that adolescents and younger adults appear to need an attachment figure who may or may not be someone who is emotionally and physically close, a confidant or in an intimate relationship with them. The attachment figure provides security to the individual because of a perceptual and emotional sense of linkage to that figure (in addition to any of the other functions). Given Weiss's reflection on the paradox of emotional isolation in later life, noted earlier, the key to understanding loneliness is therefore an understanding of how personal attachments develop and are maintained (and terminated) over the life course and particularly in later life.

## Sociological perspectives

The theoretical perspectives on loneliness discussed thus far all derive from psychology and therefore are focused at understanding and explanation located at the level of the individual. From a sociological perspective these theoretical approaches lack a key insight, namely an understanding of the social context in which individuals develop (or not) social relationships and in which they experience loneliness, isolation or social engagement. We would argue that, valuable though studies of individual-level explanations are, to try to explain and understand social engagement without an appreciation and acknowledgement of the social context is only ever going to offer a 'partial' explanation and analysis. Hence we would argue that, to understand the social relationships of older people, we need to understand both individual behaviour and the social-cultural context within which that behaviour is located.

Many of the early sociological approaches to loneliness were dominated by structural-functionalism and systems theorists for whom the behaviour of individuals, regardless of age, depends on their social environment and what society influences them into doing. These theorists therefore look for the explanations of loneliness not in the individual themselves but in particular aspects of the structure in which they live. However, such approaches overlooked the nature of interpersonal relationships and cognitive processes in their accounts of loneliness. Thus a number of functionalist sociologists followed the theoretical ideas that Emile Durkheim, writing at the end of the nineteenth century about suicide, developed about social integration and social relationships (Durkheim, 1952). Note that, yet again, the starting point for this set of theoretical propositions was a focus upon an extreme form of pathology or deviant behaviour, namely suicide. So whilst the level of explanation between social and psychological theories differs markedly they are linked in their origins of studying the deviant or 'abnormal'.

From his focus upon suicide Durkheim highlighted the key components of social integration as high levels of social interaction, social ties within a socially cohesive group and the presence of strong collective sentiments. His empirical study of European suicide rates is very important because it provided one of the earliest examples of social epidemiological investigation and established a methodological template that others have followed. Sociological investigations of social support, loneliness and social isolation have followed in this tradition with an implicit theoretical assumption that loneliness is the consequence of social isolation, which itself is a consequence of a lack of integration into social networks. This body of work in social gerontology has often been empiricist and largely atheoretical and driven by the deficit model of later life that reflects the paradigm that sees old age as a social problem.[2] Our focus is again upon the identification and articulation of the 'problems' of old age and the identification of solutions and mediating interventions. From a broadly political-economy perspective, however, theoretical ideas about social inclusion and exclusion of older people have begun to re-examine ideas of social integration and social networks and the status of older people in twenty-first-century society (Phillipson et al., 2001, 2003; Scharf et al., 2001).

However, the 'social epidemiology' tradition of work has made an important contribution to our understanding of social relationships in later life by providing answers to such questions as: Who experiences loneliness in later life? How does loneliness exhibit itself? What social contexts foster loneliness? What are the individual risk factors for loneliness? What constitutes the natural history of loneliness? What therapies or interventions, either at the group or individual level, might reduce loneliness? As these questions illustrate the focus of work generated by researchers working within this paradigm has been centred upon the negative – who is at risk of loneliness, not who does not experience this state and why or how have they 'avoided' this negative aspect of old age. Such studies have raised as many questions as they have answered for they provide little insight into the lived experience of loneliness and the definitions and understandings of loneliness, what loneliness means to older people and how they think it could be ameliorated. However, we would argue that we cannot fully answer such issues until we have answers to the fundamental theoretical questions about the way older people see loneliness and social

---

[2] We ourselves are not innocent of this criticism. See, for example, Bond, J. and Carstairs, V. (1982) *Services for the Elderly: a Survey of the Characteristics and Needs of a Population of 5,000 Old People. Scottish Health Service Studies No.42.* Edinburgh: Scottish Home and Health Department, Jones, D. A., Victor, C. R. and Vetter, N. J. (1985) 'The problem of loneliness in the elderly in the community: characteristics of those who are lonely and the factors related to loneliness', *Journal of the Royal College of General Practitioners*, 35: 136–9.

isolation in their lives. That such fundamental questions have still not been properly addressed stems largely from the dominant policy research tradition and the belief among some campaign organisations that loneliness is uniquely a problem of old age that needs to be addressed. The dominance of this view can be illustrated by the 2001/2 Help the Aged campaign to 'free our old age prisoners'. This campaign, and their recent HUGS campaign, focused on loneliness and isolation in old age. Both campaigns present an image of old age and older people as objects for pity and as individuals who are neither independent nor autonomous and who need things (in this case social participation) doing for them or to them.

## Studying social relationships in later life

Having outlined the theoretical basis for the study of social relationships in later life we now consider the methodological and measurement issues relating to the topic in general and outline the study design used in our research. We first establish some of the key principles underpinning our approach.

### Epistemological and methodological issues in loneliness research[3]

Epistemological questions are concerned with 'how do we have knowledge of the external world?' and 'what is the relationship between the knower (inquirer or researcher) and the known (or knowable)?' A key question here is whether we (the inquirer or researchers) can perceive the real world of older people and in particular the lived experiences of individual older people? An assumption of positivists and post-positivists is that because we understand what loneliness and social isolation mean for ourselves then we can define this for others and transfer across from our experiences to our research participants, regardless of differences in age, gender, ethnicity, class or biography. Critical theorists would argue that you can only understand the loneliness and social isolation of the oppressed, of which older people are an example, in one of two ways: we can either become oppressed and experience the reality of that state or by emancipating them so that they can articulate their own reality. Following this line of reasoning to

[3] This section is adapted from Bond, J. and Corner, L. (2004) *Quality of Life and Older People*. Buckingham: Open University Press, pp. 102–3.

its logical conclusion, it is only women or people who are differently abled who can describe the lived experience of being a woman or being 'disabled'. To apply this to our own area of study, then only lonely or isolated older people can offer an authentic view of this experience. As Marx so cogently recognised, this poses a challenge, as it is only those who are oppressed and who have recognised their own oppression that will be in a position to present a realist and authentic view of their life. This probably unnecessarily restricts the pool of researchers to a very small number of very unique individuals.

From a constructionist perspective we would assume that multiple realities exist and that these realities are often relative to others and can co-exist. To understand loneliness and social isolation we would need to seek an understanding of what different aspects of life mean for the individual, what is the relative value of these and what is the effect of context, particularly time and place. In the face of such complexity it is perhaps no surprise that researchers revert to a positivist or post-positivist paradigm in which their own experiences and knowledge largely dictates the nature of the questions asked. However, we argue that the 'voice' of the older person has been conspicuously absent from much research concerned with social relationships and as such we wanted to address this gap in our understanding and include this within our study. This aspiration informed the overall mixed-method design used in our study.

Methodological questions are concerned with how the inquirer should go about finding knowledge. In this case, how could we best approach the study of loneliness and isolation and our wider goal of understanding the social world of older people? How might (or might not) loneliness and social isolation have changed over time? How are they related to the individual's biography and life course? We can begin by examining the literature, identifying two major approaches to the answering of these types of question: the quantitative 'survey' and the qualitative 'in-depth' interview.

Traditional survey approaches are grounded in the researcher's definition of the situation and the extent to which these are shared by participants is unknown because of the nature of 'public accounts' (Cornwell, 1984). In the context of a research interview, the account provided by the study participant may be highly contingent upon the nature of their relationship with the interviewer, the 'interviewer effects'. This relationship will be influenced by a range of factors including the type and setting for the interview, the relative social status of the two participants in the interview and other contingencies in the life of the study participant. Context is important as well. The setting of interviews, whether it is for research purposes, appraisal interviews in the workplace or interviews with police officers during criminal investigations, affects the way that the interview is conducted and the kinds of accounts presented. Our experience of participating as subjects in such interviews suggests that we act differently when we are 'at home', in our own space (be that office or home) than we do in the more formal setting of a hospital or school, in the boss's office or in the local police station. The power of the interviewer to control and influence events increases when the setting is dictated by them and the kinds of questions they might ask.

The power of social actors during interactions of course also relates to their relative position in the social order as reflected in their gender, age, ethnic status, 'social class' as well as their roles as professional or 'officials' in society. In our complex hierarchical society the accounts we provide are highly constrained by inequalities that exist within interactions. The power of actors during interactions is also affected by the type of power which is significant to the interaction. By power we mean the ways in which 'person A could cause person B to do something which was contrary to B's desire' (French and Raven, 1968). A's dominant position during the interaction can be due to the power over rewards valued by B or 'punishments' feared by B. A's power can be legitimated by the organisational or societal context which may give her control over information, rights to access and rights to organise. In the research interview many of these different dimensions of power come into play such that the study participant becomes a 'vessel of data' (Holstein and Gubrium, 1995) rather than an active participant.

The impact of life contingencies on controlled and directed data collection about loneliness and social isolation extends the list of constraints that we have already identified for the research interview. Not least is the routine way that we respond to life events specifically and change more generally. Individual mood reflecting time and space and specific events can alter the way we respond in interviews, such that our public accounts change between interviews but have very little to do with a change in our experience of, in this case, loneliness or social isolation. Hence asking questions about patterns of engagement is inevitably problematic and, we would suggest, always subject to multiple interpretations and perspectives.

Clearly no single research approach could comprehensively address the research questions underpinning our study, which are concerned with both documenting the extent of loneliness and isolation and with understanding these concepts from the perspective of the older person and attempting to understand how the experience of these phenomena have changed over time. Our interest in examining secular changes in the extent of these social phenomena added to the complexity of our design. Given the acknowledged complexity that inevitably results from adopting a broadly constructivist approach towards research, and the differing ontological nature of our research questions, our study required a 'mixed-methods' approach.

As is described below, our study is based upon two sources of data: a fairly standard quantitative social survey and in-depth qualitative interviews. This combination of data-collection techniques is not uncommon within 'mixed-methods' research designs and our approach was to run these two study components in sequence, rather than either in parallel or via a formalised 'merging' and swapping of techniques across the differing arms of the study. The rationale for the use of a mixed-methods design was to increase the validity or trust-worthiness of our data by integrating differing perspectives to provide a stronger synthesis of our data and our understanding of the topic. However, there are particular challenges in mixed-methods research. One specific challenge is epistemological in that there often exists within mixed-methods studies incompatible and, perhaps, irreconcilable paradigm differences. Thus, by trying to coalesce the perspectives underlying the social survey and qualitative in-depth interviews (as we did in this study), we immediately face paradigm contradictions and controversies.

This chapter has provided an overview of ontological, epistemological, theoretical and methodological issues in the study of loneliness and social isolation. We contest the dominant paradigm that problematises and medicalises the experience of loneliness and social isolation and provide a broadly constructivist perspective that engages a mixed-methods design for our empirical work. In the next chapter we consider loneliness and social isolation in the broader context of older people's lives by describing patterns of social engagement of the survey population and contrasting our results with other studies and surveys completed in the UK within the past 50 years. But before we present our empirical data we finish this chapter by summarising our study methods. Our research design combines a large-scale social survey with an in-depth qualitative interview study. Each of these aspects of the study is summarised here and described more fully in the relevant chapters so that readers can evaluate and contextualise the empirical data. Before outlining our survey and qualitative interview study we consider the challenging issue of how to assess or 'measure' loneliness.

## Measuring loneliness and social isolation

Two key aspects of our research related to the identification of people who were lonely and people who were isolated and an examination of how (or how not) this had changed over time. Hence, given the issues noted above, our research question required us to attempt to measure these concepts and in a manner which would enable comparison over time with published literature and which was compatible with our constructivist position. This was no small challenge but one that was informed by the overt research objective of examining changes over time.

# Loneliness

The preceding discussion of theory and method illustrates the complexity of our research objective to measure the prevalence of loneliness. How, if at all, can we identify who is lonely and who is not? Survey researchers have used at least two different techniques in interviews to capture the reports of older people about loneliness: direct 'self-rating' question(s) and indirect scales. A common approach to the measurement of loneliness is a single question with a rating response scale. Such questions conceptualise loneliness as a one-dimensional concept. These questions, the differences which are summarised in Chapter 4, require participants to rate their current experience of loneliness. Although there are subtle differences in questions and response items in studies, each of the ratings used reflect an assumption that the variation between individuals is in the intensity of the experience rather than the nature of the experience itself. Such questions are implicitly informed by cognitive theories of loneliness that are often based upon personal assumptions. Discrepancies between desired and available relationships give rise to maladaptive patterns of thinking that can generate feelings of loneliness. Such theories underpin the use of 'self-rating' scales in the measurement of loneliness.

The emphasis in our approach to the measurement of loneliness was not to identify any subtypes of loneliness but to examine the variability of the experience across the population. For us, the single-question rating scale allowed direct comparison with other earlier British studies as well as having several attractive features. They are simple to use, appear to be highly acceptable to research participants and ask directly about feelings of loneliness. This simple scale has been found to adapt better to the oldest age groups although it does not elicit information about the amount, nature, value or meaning of loneliness, nor about its causes or consequences (Fees et al., 1999).

However, their simplicity has also been identified as a weakness. The single question assumes a common understanding of the concept by study participants and, as such, is highly culturally specific (Jylhä, 2004). Furthermore, there are potential problems with the use of the intermediate categories such as 'sometimes'. Pepper (1981) reported that respondents' interpretations of the term 'sometimes' are variable with many people understanding it to be about 20 per cent of the time, while others understanding it to mean about half the time. Such variability in interpretation is clearly problematic. Schaeffer (1991) recommends that the relative-frequency responses currently used in many scales be replaced by absolute-frequency responses, such as 'everyday' or 'once a week'. By using absolute-frequency response options, comparisons between groups would reflect real differences in the prevalence of loneliness and not be caused by differences in how different groups interpret the relative-frequency response options. In addition, 'self-rating scales' have very limited psychometric data to attest to their robustness. The earliest use of this simple 'self-rating' scale that we have identified is in the study reported by Sheldon (1948) but it is not clear if he devised this question or what, if any, tests were undertaken to establish the validity and reliability of the measure.

But the key objection to the use of single-question self-rating scales to measure the extent of loneliness is that they will not elicit a 'true' response: they will generate only a 'publicly acceptable' response. Although single questions about loneliness may exhibit face validity they could be answered in an 'ego-defensive manner' (Solano, 1980). 'Self-rating' scales require respondents to 'admit' their loneliness and so potential respondents may down play their responses for fear of compromising their sense of self-worth during the interview. However, other approaches are not without their problems. Multiple-question scales can also elicit 'socially desirable responses'. For example, the Social and Emotional Loneliness Scale for Adults (SELSA) used by Treacy et al. (2005) in Ireland requires respondents to answer questions such as 'In the last year I felt alone when I was with my family' and 'In the last year there was no one in my family that I could depend upon for support and encouragement'. These are challenging questions which are highly likely to elicit response bias.

In the sense that perceived loneliness is an 'attitude', psychometricians and survey researchers have strongly argued the limitations of the single-question self-rating scale and the preferred technique accepted as the 'gold standard' is the use of a number of scaled items in a scale of loneliness. Attitudinal questions are extremely sensitive to changes in wording, emphasis, context, response categories and the mood of the individual and, therefore, for single questions it is difficult to estimate their reliability or validity. Reliability refers to the purity and consistency of a measure and to its repeatability in both time and place. We would wish to know the probability that our single question obtains the same results again if the question were repeated. In contrast, validity is concerned with whether our single question measures what we believe it measures. Sets of questions or attitude scales made up of a number of statements or items are preferred because the vagaries of question wording may vary across scale items and thus any biases may cancel each other out. By using sets of questions, provided they all relate to the same attitude, the stable components can be maximised while reducing the instability of individual questions.

The use of multiple-question scaling techniques makes the assessment of reliability straightforward and easy to report using inter-item analysis (Cronbach, 1951). Validity remains difficult to assess although the questions or items used can be investigated for face validity by checking that they make sense to survey participants using cognitive interviewing methods (Willis, 2005). Thus the assumption underlying this approach is that there is such a thing as a 'true' attitude, that the 'attitude' is relatively stable, that the underlying attitude is common to all the items in the scale and that the construct being researched has the same meaning for all participants. As indicated previously, this is a highly positively orientated approach which presumes that there is a 'true' prevalence of loneliness that exists and which such measures will capture.

It is not our aim to provide a comprehensive review of multiple-questions loneliness scales and their psychometric properties. In 1982 when Russell reviewed measures of loneliness only two existed within the published literature: the UCLA Loneliness Scale (an example of a single-dimensional measure) (Russell, 1982) developed at the University of California and widely used in European settings, and the de Jong-Gierveld loneliness scale (an example of a multidimensional measure) (de Jong-Gierveld and Raadschelders, 1982) developed in the United States but modified and widely used in the Netherlands and other European settings. Both scales have been used to assess loneliness in all age groups.

## The University of California Los Angeles loneliness scale

The UCLA loneliness scale was developed predominantly with young people and college students and distinguishes between social and emotional loneliness (Weiss, 1973). This is an interesting observation since the predominant stereotype is that loneliness is especially a feature of later life, yet the most influential scale in North America was not developed with this population in mind. This partly reflects the particular interests of social psychologists who have studied loneliness as a personality trait or as a state-related entity that has a transient response to social circumstances.

The assumption behind the single-dimension UCLA loneliness scale is that there are common themes in the experience of loneliness irrespective of the possible causes of loneliness. Thus, the older person who has just experienced a significant loss, such as the death of their life-long partner, is assumed to be experiencing loneliness in the same way as a life-long 'loner' or introvert who has never established meaningful social relations with other human beings. The scale was developed in response to the absence of a psychometrically acceptable multiple-question scale to measure 'loneliness' in individuals. The developers

---

**Box 2.2  The 10 item UCLA Loneliness Scale**

1. _____ I am unhappy doing so many things alone.

2. _____ I don't have anybody to talk to.

3. _____ I can't tolerate being so alone.

4. _____ Nobody really understands me.

5. _____ I often wait for people to call or write.

6. _____ I feel completely alone.

7. _____ I'm unable to reach out and communicate with those around me.

8. _____ I feel starved for company.

9. _____ It is difficult for me to make friends.

10._____ I feel shut out and exluded by others.

These are scored never (0), sometimes (2) often (3) and always (4)

*Source:* Russell (1982)

---

sought to create a tool that would be psychometrically adequate, easily administered and generally available and which could be used in a variety of populations and settings. The original UCLA loneliness scale comprised 20 items with the revised scale consisting of 10 items (see Box 2.2). The scale was developed using items from other studies and unpublished scales, including the Belcher Extended Loneliness Scale. It was first administered to a group of student volunteers. Further development comprised the rewording of items and the development of a self-labelling index with a separate group of volunteer students. A second study using a representative sample of college students compared the UCLA loneliness scale with the self-labelling index and other aspects of a student's life world. The final scale reported generally acceptable measures of internal consistency, discriminant validity and correlation with other similar measures and has been subjected to a confirmatory factor analysis in a student population (Hartshorne, 1993). It is also reported as being responsive to change and its widespread use means that there are population norms available for a variety of different populations and countries.

There remain limitations with the scale. Respondents are required to classify their response and the ambiguous 'sometimes' category is present as one of the response options. The scoring scale used is an interval scale that assumes that 'always' is four times worse than 'never'. The cultural and social context within which this scale was developed is clearly evident in the scale items such as 'I often wait for people to call or write', 'I feel completely alone', 'I'm unable to reach out and communicate with those around me'. Consequently, there are inherent problems in translating a measure derived from North America and tested and validated with college students to the UK and an older population. More recently a short version of the UCLA scale consisting of three items has been developed in response to the need to be able to incorporate the scale into wide-ranging social surveys (Hughes et al., 2004) such as the US Health and Retirement survey and the portmanteau telephone-based surveys used in the United States and increasingly elsewhere. This scale consists of three items and uses a simplified set of response categories. The items are: (a) How often do you feel you lack companionship? (b) How often do you feel left out? and (c) How often do you feel isolated from others? With responses on a three-point scale – hardly ever, some of the time and often. A four-item version of this scale is used in the English Longitudinal Study of Ageing (ELSA) (Banks et al., 2006) with the additional question, How often do you feel in tune with the people around you? The initial data from ELSA are presented in terms of responses to the four questions rather than as an overall index which limits its utility for this volume.

## The de Jong-Gierveld loneliness scale

The alternative multidimensional approach sees loneliness as a complex phenomenon, the essence of which cannot be captured by a single-dimensional global scale. Rather than focus on communalities underlying the experiences of loneliness for all individuals this approach attempts to differentiate between the diverse causes underlying the experience of loneliness among different groups of individuals and the goal of the developers is to differentiate the varying types of loneliness. Loneliness is conceptualised as a multidimensional concept. A good example of this latter approach is the multidimensional measure of loneliness developed over many years by de Jong-Gierveld (de Jong-Gierveld and Raadschelders, 1982) and reflected in her definition of loneliness quoted above.

The development of the de Jong-Gierveld scale of loneliness is described by van Tilburg and de Leeuw (1991). Study participants (N = 114) were invited to write about their experiences of loneliness and the resulting compositions were content analysed. From this analysis scale items were constructed and administered in a small pilot study (N = 59). A revised set of items was administered in semi-structured interviews to a further 556 men and women. Further revision of items was thought necessary and a revised scale was administered in a self-completed questionnaire to 1600 people as part of a structured interview within a national governmental survey in the Netherlands. The scale is also reported to meet the criteria of the dichotomous logistic Rasch model (de Jong-Gierveld and Kamphuis, 1985) and a new six-item version has just been validated (de Jong-Gierveld and Van Tilburg, 2006).

Three dimensions can be distinguished (de Jong-Gierveld, 1987). The first concerns the feelings and emotions associated with the absence of an intimate attachment, for example feelings of emptiness and abandonment. We could describe this as a kind of emotional deprivation or perhaps in Townsend's language social desolation (Townsend and Tunstall, 1968). For de Jong-Gierveld this is the core dimension of the concept of loneliness (de Jong-Gierveld, 1998: 74). The second dimension represents their current feelings about loneliness. For example, does the individual interpret their loneliness as being hopeless or something which is treatable or transient? Or, do they blame themselves or others for their loneliness? The third component describes a range of emotional experiences including sorrow, sadness and feelings of shame, guilt or frustration. Items included in the scale are shown in Box 2.3.

The de Jong-Gierveld Scale of Loneliness represents a paradigmatic example of the post-positivist perspective and is well grounded in the established psychological theories of loneliness. But the scale itself appears to conflate different emotional experiences that might themselves be due to factors other than the absence of an intimate attachment including factors that influence anxiety, depression and personal and psychological well-being. Of course mental health and well-being have been shown to be strongly associated with loneliness (and social isolation) (Bowling et al., 1989).

---

**Box 2.3 The de Jong-Gierveld Scale of Loneliness**

There is always someone that I can talk to about my day to day problems.
I miss having a really close friend.
I experience a general sense of emptiness.
There are plenty of people that I can lean on in case of trouble.
I miss the pleasure of the company of others.
I feel my circle of friends and acquaintances is too limited.
There are many people that I can count on completely.
There are enough people are feel close to.
I miss having people around.
I often feel rejected.
I can call my friends whenever I need them.

*Source:* van Tilburg and de Leeuw (1991: 72)

---

## The Social and Emotional Loneliness Scale for Adults

Another multidimensional scale used with adults is the Social and Emotional Loneliness Scale for Adults (SELSA) (Treacy et al., 2005). This is a 37-item instrument that differentiates social and emotional loneliness (see Box 2.4). The short form of this measure consists of 15 items measuring three components: family loneliness, romantic loneliness and social loneliness (Di Tommaso et al., 2004).

## Wenger Loneliness Scale

None of the multiple dimensional measures of loneliness that we have considered have been developed on the UK (older) population. The nearest we have to a 'home-grown' loneliness scale is the composite measure developed by Wenger (1983) based upon her research in north Wales. The Wenger scale is very rarely used by other researchers and certainly does not have the popularity of either the de Jong scale or the UCLA scale. Indeed Mayers et al. (2005) suggest that 80 per cent of studies of loneliness now use the UCLA measure. Although it is not clear how this statement was arrived at, it is clear that the UCLA scale is very widely used. This suggests some indirect evidence that the use of the UCLA loneliness scale offers insights into a valid social phenomena. The Wenger index is an example of how individual researchers develop their own scales to suit the particular research context within which

---

**Box 2.4  The SELSA-S loneliness scale**

**Social subscale**

In the last year I felt part of a group of friends.
In the last year my friends understood me.
In the last year I didn't have a friend.
In the last year I was able to depend on my friends for help.
In the last year I didn't have a friend or friends who cared about me.

**Family subscale**

In the last year I felt alone when I was with my family.
In the last year there was no one in my family that I could depend on for emotional support.
In the last year I felt close to my family.
In the last year I felt part of my family.
In the last year my family really cared about me.

**Romantic subscale**

In the last year I had a partner/friend with whom I shared my thoughts and feelings.
In the last year I had a partner/friend who gave me the support and encouragement I needed.
In the last year I wish I had a closer relationship.
In the last year I had a partner who made me happy.
In the last year I would have liked a closer relationship with another person.

*Source:* Treacy et al. (2005)

---

they are working: in this case, a rural area of north Wales with a specific cultural milieu. The eight items included in this scale are shown in Box 2.5 and are very different from the content of the other two scales, focusing much more upon network links than internal feelings of isolation.

The development and acceptance of theories of loneliness, and the measurement of the phenomena within populations has been hampered by the fact that loneliness is often masked by other clinical syndromes. For example, there is a strong association between loneliness and depression (Adams et al., 2004). There is an obvious and consistent link between loneliness and depression – indeed depression indices often include questions about loneliness. Depression is a

---

**Box 2.5 The Wenger loneliness index**

All items have a seven-point response format ranging from strongly agree to strongly disagree.

Feels lonely much of the time.
Does not see enough of friends/relatives.
Does not meet enough people.
Has no confidant.
Wishes for more friends.
Has no one to ask favours.
Has no real friends living near by.
Spent Christmas alone and lonely.

*Source:* Wenger (1983)

---

problem that often accompanies loneliness and depressive symptomotology such as withdrawal, anxiety, lack of motivation and sadness both mimic and mask the manifestations of loneliness. In such cases, people are often treated for depression without considering the possibility that loneliness may be a contributing and sustaining factor in their condition. Consequently, loneliness has often been subsumed under depression, anxiety or as social isolation rather than being recognised as a distinct problem.

The scales described above, with the exception of the Wenger loneliness scale, are strongly rooted within the psychological tradition of loneliness research and have an explicit empiricist and positivist foundation. However, as we have already argued, such theoretical perspectives, and their associated measures, do not embrace the broader social context nor acknowledge the potentially multiple perspectives and understandings that exist. As we indicated with the single-question rating scale, questions and their responses do not offer any insight into the nature, value, meaning, causes or consequences of loneliness. Illumination of these issues was an important component of our study.

In the present study a mixed-methods approach to self-reported subjective loneliness was adopted so that we could specifically address these issues. We have noted the problems of working with multiple paradigms. Since our perspective is broadly social constructionist it was appropriate within the context of a population-based social survey to stay within the accepted canons of the method and to ask a single question about how often the survey participant experienced loneliness.

There are, of course, many limitations of this approach and we are exposed to critics from both constructionists and positivists. From social constructionist and qualitative methods perspectives a single, structured question is clearly inadequate and does not allow the participant to reflect sufficiently on either the meaning of the concept or the meaning of loneliness to the individual. Responses are likely to reflect the 'public voice' (Cornwell, 1984; Corner, 1999; Bond and Corner, 2004) of participants rather than their 'private voice'. Loneliness is a potentially stigmatising concept. Are those who experience this state likely to report this within an interview situation and thereby risk 'damaging' their personal sense of worth and evaluation by the interviewer?

From the post-positivist and survey methods perspectives a single question does not meet the psychometric principles of attitude measurement and scale construction noted earlier and which are so important within the quantitative research tradition. We justify our use of a single question on four counts, which reflect a combination of pragmatism in the face of 'real world' constraints and the nature of our research questions. First, the single question used, although open to different understandings and cognitive interpretations by participants, does present an everyday life concept that is routinely used in daily interactions, by the media, by campaigning groups and politicians. It has a common-sense appeal that makes it practical and relevant to ask and 'easy' for participants to answer. Within the structured interview this question was embedded within the broader context of seeking the participant's experience of later life. Second, as with all surveys there were constraints on the amount of data that we could capture. Third, we were keen to be able to make historical and, where possible, cross-cultural comparisons with surveys undertaken in the 1950s, 1960s and 1970s. For this purpose the importance of using exactly the same questions has been well documented. Fourth, by taking a mixed-method approach we were able to unpick the meaning of the question to participants who also participated in follow-up qualitative interviews. Within these interviews we were able to take a traditional social constructionist approach to investigating the lived experience of older people and the meaning and understanding they gave to issues such as loneliness and isolation. Hence our analysis and interpretation of responses to the 'single-item' question was informed by our qualitative data collection as the 'mixed-method' approach suggests.

## Social isolation

Social isolation has generally been 'measured' in three similar but contrasting ways: by counting social contacts, by counting social activities and by describing social networks. The early UK community studies followed the lead of Townsend (1957) and Tunstall (1966) who asked respondents a number of questions about contact with extended family members, neighbours and friends within specific temporal reference periods, usually the last week. Participation in social activities provided a natural extension to this approach, which in turn was used in the description of network types (Wenger, 1984). Each of these related approaches has its strengths and weaknesses.

In the measurement of social contacts, the inclusion and exclusion of particular kin relationships and wider social relationships such as friends and neighbours was specific to different studies and researchers. The quality of interactions was rarely evaluated but assumptions were clearly made about the importance of certain relationships, such as the husband-wife and mother-daughter relationships, over other relationships and of the primacy of direct contacts, although at the time the empirical evidence for these evaluations was limited. A contextual feature of these early studies was the focus on physical contact encapsulated in the question 'How often do you see X?' Other methods of contact, increasingly prevalent in the twenty-first century, such as phone conversations or internet communication via email or on-line conversations were not included (for obvious reasons) in the earlier studies. But there appears to be a time lag in the inclusion of such technologically induced social change in later studies measuring social isolation. It is not until the national study reported by Hunt (1978) that the telephone was asked about as a method of promoting and maintaining social relationships rather than as a means of 'emergency' contact. But from a common-sense perspective, counting social contacts, however you define contact, probably provides an objective measure of social contact as long as the quality of relationships, duration of relationships and interaction and the weighting of significant relationships is not seen as an essential feature of social isolation. Hence, in our study we asked participants to report their frequency of contact with family, friends and relatives via a variety of mediums using questions derived from the 1998 General Household Survey (Bridgwood et al., 2000), although we could not distinguish where contacts had taken place (see Chapter 3 for details of questions). This offers the strength of enabling us to locate our survey within a broader context, both by enabling us to consider the generalisability of our findings and by enabling us to address cross-generational levels of engagement. However, as our questions collect responses in terms of categories or broad levels of contacts rather than absolute numbers, this limits the precision of any calculated 'social isolation' index composed solely of these variables.

Although the counting of social activities has also been included in the assessment of social isolation there has been less adherence to this approach by survey researchers. Participation in specific social activities and changes in participation over time have clearly been of interest (Bridgwood, 2000). However, the challenge of making qualitative judgements about, for example, the relative contribution television watching or visiting the local pub has to social isolation has been avoided in recognition of the complexity and inappropriateness of making such judgements. The counting of social activities, particularly social activities outside the home such as church participation, however, has become an important feature of research on the social networks of older people. As we have already noted, the types, location and nature of the activities used in such studies reflects broader social changes and moral judgements about what are considered 'proper' or appropriate activities for older people. In our survey we included a range of ativities that have 'traditionally' been included in such studies such as walking and gardening but we also included items such as eating out and visiting the threatre. Full details are provided in Chapter 3.

Given the ubiquitous use of the concept in epidemiological and social research, there have been surprisingly few coherent attempts to measure the social networks of older people (Glass et al., 1997), although different classifications of network types have emerged (Wenger, 1984 and 1989; Antonucci and Akiyama, 1987; van Sonderen,

1990; Litwin, 1995). There has been much more emphasis on the measurement of social support in which social contact and social network are important contributions. Although social support is a relevant concept to consider when investigating social isolation, the over-arching emphasis of the social support literature is on the pro- vision of help and support to older people with physical or mental incapacity rather than with notions of isolation and loneliness. We therefore focus here on the aspects of social relationships that relate most closely to the measurement of social isolation rather than the more usual focus upon the 'supportive' functions of networks.

## Study design

As we have already indicated we used a mixed-methods design that comprised a national social survey and in-depth qualitative interviews with a sample of participants responding to the national survey.

### The social survey

We refer to the social survey as the ESRC GO survey or, more per- sonally, our survey! The ESRC GO survey used the 2001 Office of National Statistics (ONS) *Omnibus Survey* of households in Great Britain as a vehicle for sampling a representative group of older people living in private households. The *Omnibus Survey* is a face-to-face interview survey that is conducted monthly or bi-monthly with approximately 2000 people aged 16 years or over. It randomly selects 30 addresses in each of 100 randomly selected 'postal sectors', which provide a broadly representative sample of adults resident in private households in Britain. Independent researchers can purchase specific modules or questions on the survey, or use it to identify eligible research participants. Respondents aged 65 or over participating in the *Omnibus Survey* (the index interview) were invited to participate in a second interview that focused on quality of life (for further details see Bowling et al., 2002; Ayis et al., 2003; Bowling, 2005; Victor et al., 2005b) and included our questions on loneliness, social isolation, social participation and related factors. The quality-of-life module also comprised detailed questions on quality of life, health status and dis- ability. Along with standard demographic and socio-economic data collected in the *Omnibus Survey* index interviews we also had access to all the data generated in the quality-of-life module. To control for seasonality and to obtain sufficient statistical power, all older respondents to the April, September and November 2000 and January 2001 waves of the *Omnibus Survey* were invited to participate in a second interview. Those who agreed were re-interviewed two months after the index interview.

The data captured in both interviews allow a post-positivist interpretation of the characteristics of older people's lives and analyses that investigate the associations between participant characteristics and their reported experience of loneliness and social isolation. As with any survey, the interpretation of the analyses is only as robust as the quality of the original survey in terms of the operationalisation of concepts such as loneliness and social isolation and the representativeness of the sample. At a first glance the 999 older people participating in the quality-of-life module appear to be a fairly large sample. We need to remind our readers that the ESRC GO survey only includes older people living at home (private households) in the community and does not include older people living in non-private households, particularly nursing homes or care homes. Our analysis therefore does not reflect the characteristics of people living in supported environments where the lived experience of residents may be rather different from older people living in their own homes.

Our survey is also subject to a possibly large non-response bias because of the staged sampling strategy we used to obtain our sample of older people. Table 2.1 reports the cumulative response rates to the *Omnibus Survey* and the ESRC GO survey. In the *Omnibus Survey* interviews were only achieved with 62 per cent of eligible households; a not particularly robust response rate. Of these interviews, 1598 were with people aged 65 or over. Eighty-three per cent agreed to participate in ESRC GO but with subsequent sample attrition the final response rate was only 63 per cent; again not a particularly robust response rate. The cumulative impact of the non-response in both surveys is difficult to estimate and we therefore express some concerns about the representativeness of our survey participants.

## Characteristics of our sample

So how representative are our survey participants? To judge this we need to compare the characteristics of participants with the

**Table 2.1** Response rates to Omnibus Survey and ESRC GO survey

|  | Number | % |
| --- | --- | --- |
| *Omnibus Survey response* | | |
| Selected addresses | 12,000 | 100 |
| Ineligible addresses | 1,099 | 9 |
| Eligible addresses | 10,909 | 100 |
| Refusals | 3,034 | 28 |
| Non-contacts | 1,164 | 11 |
| Interviews achieved | 6,711 | 62 |
| Omnibus surveys interviews achieved with people aged | | |
| 65 years or over | 1,598 | 100 |
| Agreement to re-interview for ESRC GO survey | 1,323 | 83 |
| Refused re-interview for ESRC GO survey | 275 | 17 |
| *ESRC GO survey response* | | |
| Selected individuals | 1,323 | 100 |
| Ineligible individuals | 24 | 2 |
| Eligible individuals | 1,299 | 100 |
| Refusals on recontact | 243 | 19 |
| Non-contacts during ESRC GO fieldwork | 57 | 4 |
| Interviews achieved[+] | 999 | 77[¥] |

*Notes:* + Includes seven partial interviews.
¥ This represents a response rate of 63 per cent for the 1,598 Omnibus Survey participants aged 65 years or over.
*Sources:* Bowling et al. (2002), Bowling (2005) Table 2.1.

characteristics of participants from the Census and other studies and surveys. For the purpose of our analyses we should examine those characteristics that have been shown to be associated with loneliness or social isolation. Previous research has identified a plethora of variables that are associated with loneliness or social isolation (see Wenger et al., 1996; de Jong-Gierveld, 1998; Victor et al., 2000). These can be grouped into five sets of factors or resource groups including:

1. Demographic factors (e.g. age, gender, household composition and marital status).

2. 'Life events' (e.g. bereavement, widowhood, onset of illness).

3. Health resources (e.g. chronic poor physical or mental health, sensory impairments, falls, self-rated health and health expectations).

4. Social resources (e.g. availability of family and friends, social contacts and social participation).

5. Material resources (e.g. home ownership, access to car and educational qualifications).

These variables are all included within our survey. We also included novel factors not previously examined in studies of social relationships including: ethnicity, material circumstances, neighbourhood quality and newly emerging means of social engagement such as email. (But not text messaging, which at the time we were designing the study in 1999 had not been recognised, particularly among older people, as such a widespread form of communication as is now established). As Bowling (2005) has also documented, many of these characteristics are similar to the general population (see Tables 2.2a and b). For example, the proportion of our participants living alone or living with a chronic illness, two key variables associated with loneliness or social isolation, is comparable to the general population: 33 per cent of our participants lived alone and 42 per cent reported a long-standing limiting illness compared with 37 per cent and 42 per cent of participants in the 1998 *General Household Survey* (Bridgwood, 2000). Further evaluation of the characteristics of our survey participants suggests that the study population is broadly representative of those older people living at home in the community with the exception of an over-representation of people who were widowed (see Victor et al., 2005b).

Although we can claim representativeness of our data, the sample size is still too small to report robustly on some key groups within the older population. For example, the absolute numbers of the very old, those aged 85 years and over, are small with only 72 in this age category. This obviously limits the degree to which we can undertake specific analyses of the very old. Similarly we had only 20 people (2 per cent) who defined themselves as being from an ethnic minority group. Again this reflects the national profile but the small numbers do not enable us to make any specific observations about social relationships with the population of minority elders. This would require a special study which focuses upon these groups or the use of 'over sampling' to

**Table 2.2a** Demographic characteristics of ESRC GO survey participants and General Household Survey 2001 (weighted estimates)

| | ESRC GO[1] | | GHS 2001[2] | |
| | Weighted Number[+] | Unweighted number[‡] | %[¥] | % |
|---|---|---|---|---|
| *Gender* | | | | |
| Men | 519 | (475) | 52 | 44 |
| Women | 480 | (524) | 48 | 56 |
| *Age group (years)* | | | | |
| 65–74 | 624 | (582) | 62 | 55 |
| 75–84 | 314 | (343) | 31 | 36 |
| 85 or over | 61 | (72) | 6 | 9 |
| *Marital status* | | | | |
| Single | 56 | (79) | 6 | 6 |
| Married/cohabiting | 616 | (460) | 62 | 55 |
| Divorced/separated | 52 | (72) | 5 | } 39 |
| Widowed | 275 | (388) | 28 | |
| *Ethnic status* | | | | |
| White | 983 | (984) | 98 | * |
| Black Caribbean | 7 | (7) | 1 | * |
| Other | 8 | (7) | 1 | * |
| *Household composition* | | | | |
| Single-person household | 313 | (469) | 31 | 36 |
| Married/cohabiting | 548 | (441) | 55 | 48 |
| Other | 139 | (89) | 14 | 16 |

*Notes:* + Weighted number to adjust for household size
‡ Raw frequencies (unweighted)
¥ Percentages do not always round to 100 because of rounding
* Not available
*Sources:* 1. Bowling (2005); 2. General Household Survey (2001)

ensure there were sufficient members of the target population to undertake the required analysis to draw meaningful conclusions.

Our colleague Ann Bowling in her book *Ageing Well* (Bowling, 2005) has provided an extensive description of the study group. Here we have focused upon the key demographic characteristics previously linked with loneliness and isolation. In Table 2.3 we make comparisons with

**Table 2.2b** Resource characteristics of ESRC GO Survey participants and General Household Survey 2001

| | ESRC GO[1] | | GHS 2001[2] | |
| | Weighted Number[+] | Unweighted number[‡] | %[¥] | % |
| --- | --- | --- | --- | --- |
| *Age left full-time education* | | | | |
| Under 15 years | 486 | (500) | 49 | * |
| 15 to 18 years | 406 | (399) | 41 | * |
| 18 years or over | 103 | (96) | 10 | * |
| *Gross annual income* | | | | |
| *before tax* | | | | |
| Less than £4160 | 218 | (202) | 23 | |
| £4160 < £6240 | 223 | (248) | 23 | |
| £6240 < £9360 | 212 | (221) | 22 | |
| £9360 < £17680 | 202 | (190) | 21 | |
| £17680 or more | 97 | (89) | 10 | |
| *Housing tenure* | | | | |
| Owns home outright | 692 | (660) | 69 | |
| Owns home, mortgage or loan | 68 | (62) | 7 | |
| Rents, local authority or | | | | |
| housing association | 199 | (236) | 20 | |
| Rents privately | 39 | (40) | 4 | |

*Notes:* + Weighted number to adjust for household size
  ‡ Raw frequencies (unweighted)
  ¥ Percentages do not always round to 100 because of rounding
  * Not available
*Sources:* 1. Bowling (2005); 2. General Household Survey (2001)

the index studies that we wish to make reference to in establishing cohort patterns of loneliness and isolation. Examination of Table 2.3 reveals that the composition of our sample is very different from that described in ealier studies. These studies had a greater preponderance of women and people who were widowed. For example, 70 per cent of Sheldon's and Townsend's respondents were women and 45 per cent were widowed. This is only partly accounted for by the inclusion of women aged 60 or over compared with men aged 65 or over, reflecting the differential retirement ages. Table 2.3 confirms the picture described in more detail by Victor (2005) of increasing male survival into old age and a resultant 'decrease' in the gender imbalance in later life, although a higher proportion of women are surviving beyond the age of 90 (Office of National Statistics, 2005). This is also reflected in the greater percentage of older people remaining married in old age. In Sheldon's survey 44 per cent of respondents were married compared with 62 per cent in our survey. Comparison across surveys also reflects the influence of changing social norms; Sheldon did not include the category of 'divorced' in his study. These demographic changes are important when considering cohort-based analyses of loneliness as gender, marital status, advanced age and living alone have all been associated with loneliness. Hence any changes in reported prevalence of loneliness may simply reflect differences in the study population composition. On the basis of the data presented we would expect rates of loneliness to be lower in our study.

One of the key changes in the demographic profile of our survey participants with the generation of older people 50 years earlier is in the relative and absolute numbers of people living alone. This is clearly evident in Table 2.3 where the percentage has increased from one in twenty to over one in three. This is, of course, a phenomenon not exclusive to older people as single-person households have become more common at all ages of the population; 17 per cent of people aged 16 and over now live alone compared with nine per cent in 1973 (Fido et al., 2006).

Living alone is a factor that has been demonstrated to have a statistical association with the pathological dimensions of social relationships, loneliness and isolation (Wenger et al., 1996). It is the increase in the percentage of older people living alone that has fuelled much of the stereotype about the social neglect, isolation and loneliness of older people. Indeed, the increasing number of people of all ages living alone is a source of concern to commentators on social cohesion. However, we must be wary of drawing a causal relationship between what is simply an association and to evaluate living alone as a purely negative experience. As one of our participants in the qualitative interviews commented:

> Purely out of choice. I wouldn't want anybody to live with me. I'm ... I suppose living on my own since 1972 I've got very selfish, because I do what I want to do, when I want to do it. And I buy what I want when I

**Table 2.3** Composition of the study population and main comparison samples (percentages)

|  | Sheldon 1948 | Townsend 1957 | Shanas et al. 1968 | Hunt 1978 | Bond and Carstairs 1982 | ESRC GO survey |
|---|---|---|---|---|---|---|
| Male | 32 | 31 | 40 | 40 | 39 | 47 |
| *Age* | | | | | | |
| 60–64 | 16 | | | | | |
| 65–74 | 54 | | 64 | 66 | 66 | 62 |
| 75+ | 30 | | 36 | 33 | 34 | 38 |
| *Marital status* | | | | | | |
| Married | 44 | 43 | 48 | 52 | 52 | 62 |
| Widowed | 39 | | 41 | 38 | 34 | 27 |
| Divorced | – | | | 2 | – | 6 |
| Single | 10 | | 11 | 8 | 11 | 5 |
| Lives alone | 10 | 25 | 22 | 30 | 32 | 33 |

*Sources:* Sheldon (1948), Townsend (1957), Shanas et al. (1968), Hunt (1978), Bond and Carstairs (1982).

want to buy it, and I don't have to ask anybody. If I want a new carpet I go any buy it. When I was younger I would have said yes I would have liked to have met someone else but it wasn't to be. And I'm not discontent with the life I lead now [305: 5: 34–40].

Overall Table 2.3 illustrates how the composition of the older population changes over time and, therefore, the experience of later life may also be presumed to be dynamic. We shall return to some of these themes in subsequent chapters.

## The qualitative study

The qualitative interview study used the quantitative survey as a sampling frame. Participants were selected using purposeful sampling methods. The reported stories provide a rich source of data about the social world of older people at the beginning of the twenty-first century and afford potential explanations for some of the associations and statistical trends observed in the analyses of the survey data. They also provide considerable insights into the lives and activities of older people. Our intention was to use the two different sources of data to complement each other and to provide a fuller picture of the social world of older people.

For the qualitative study 68 participants were sampled. Of these 15 refused (six for health reasons, six did not state a reason and three reported that they were 'over-researched'), six were not contactable, one had moved and one potential participant was sampled by Gabriel and Bowling (2004a) for their qualitative study of older people. The number of participants in the qualitative study is 45: a participation rate of 66 per cent. Participants were sampled theoretically from participants in our survey using the following characteristics: geographical location, age, gender, ethnicity, socio-economic status, living arrangements and type of housing. Completed interviews were conducted with 18 men and 27 women aged between 65 and 90 years. Their characteristics are summarised in Table 2.4 and compared with the survey participants. Although the qualitative sample was not intended to be representative, we can see that the sample contains a higher proportion of those who were widowed and living alone than in the survey.

**Table 2.4** Characteristics (%) of the participants in the qualitative study (n = 45)

| Variable | Qualitative study (%) | Main survey (%) |
| --- | --- | --- |
| Male | 39 | 47 |
| Aged 75+ | 41 | 38 |
| Widowed | 37 | 27 |
| Living alone | 46 | 33 |
| Never lonely | 52 | 61 |
| More lonely than 10 years ago | 35 | 23 |

Two options for the sampling of participants were considered: 1) by relationship with isolation and loneliness, or 2) by geographical area, which was the method used by Tunstall (1966). Our initial pilot study in south London (Victor et al., 2002) suggested that the development of theoretical sampling associated with loneliness or social isolation would be problematic because of small cell sizes. This strategy, however, was used successfully by Iredell et al. (2003) in a limited geographical area of the city of Perth, Western Australia. For pragmatic reasons five areas in England were initially selected to replicate the sampling frame of Tunstall (1966) with the intention of interviewing ten participants in each area. These were: the South Coast (typical retirement areas), East Anglia, the South West (rural and retirement areas), the East Midlands and the North East (urban and industrial areas). Following the pilot study (Victor et al., 2002), London (a multicultural metropolitan area) and Surrey (an affluent commuter belt) were added to provide a broader range of areas and reflect the emergence of two groups unlikely to have been very numerous when Tunstall undertook his study: ethnic minority elders and the experience of growing old within a multicultural area; and the 'affluent elders'. Difficulties in accessing people meant that we were unable to complete ten interviews in each area (see Table 2.5).

**Table 2.5** Number of completed in-depth interviews in sampled areas (qualitative study)

| Area | N |
| --- | --- |
| South Coast | 6 |
| East Anglia | 7 |
| South West | 10 |
| East Midlands | 7 |
| North East | 3 |
| London | 7 |
| Surrey | 5 |

All of the interviews were conducted in the home of the participant. In five of the interviews partners of the sampled participant were present and took part in answering the questions, and in the remaining 40 the participant was either alone in the house or their partner remained in another room whilst the interview took place. The interviews took between 30 and 90 minutes to complete with an average length of approximately 60 minutes.

An interview topic guide was generated following our experience of the pilot study (See Box 2.6).

**BOX 2.6 The qualitative interview guide**

◆ How old are you?

◆ Are you married/single/widowed/divorced?

◆ Do you live alone/with family/with friends?

◆ How long have you lived in this house/area?

◆ Do you have any children?
   If so do they live locally?

◆ Do you have any pets?

◆ Describe an average week day.
   What do you do?
   Where do you go?
   Who do you see?
   Are you happy with the way you spend your time?
   If not, why not?

◆ Do weekends differ from weekdays?
   Do you do different things?
   Do you see different people?

◆ How often do you see members of your family?
   Are you happy with the amount you see of your family?
   What do you do when you are together?
   How do you stay in contact with them?
   (visit, travel, phone, letter, email)

◆ How often do you see your friends?
   Are you happy with the amount you see your friends?
   What do you do when you are together?
   Do you have a group of friends?
   Do you travel to see people?
   How do you stay in contact with friends?
   Do you visit a day centre or club?

◆ Do you have a close friend or family member that you could turn to for support if you needed it?

◆ Would you rather spend time:
   On you own?
   With family?
   With friends?

- Do you ever feel lonely?
  Do you enjoy spending your time alone?
  Is loneliness a problem for older people?
- How would you define loneliness?
- Do you ever feel isolated?
- Has this changed as you have got older?
- How would you define isolation?
- Has the way you spend your time changed as you have got older?
  If so how?
  If so why?
  If not would you like it to?
- Has your social life changed since you retired?
  If so how?
- Does your health/mobility/age affect the way in which you spend your time?
- Is there anything that you would change about the way you spend your time?
- Is there anything you would like to do but can't?
- Is there anything you would like access to but do not have?

Here we summarise the key areas of questioning, which were clustered around a series of themes:

- The perceived importance of social interaction.

- The role of loss within people's experiences of loneliness.

- The temporal nature of loneliness.

- The presence of different pathways into loneliness.

- The conceptual framework employed when defining loneliness.

- Factors that influence whether or not people experience loneliness.

- The importance of citizenship and political participation.

## Analysis of qualitative interviews

All of the interviews were audio-recorded and transcribed in full. Each transcript was coded according to a thematic framework developed during the pilot study and the coding of the first few transcripts. Summary sheets were then produced for each transcript highlighting the key theme and factors causing loneliness. The three authors independently coded a sample of transcripts. The identified themes were compared to ensure that the themes emerging from the data were consistently highlighted by each of the coders. Few important differences in the application of the thematic coding frame were identified.

Throughout the book we use transcript material to illustrate and provide a deeper understanding of the survey data. Extracts of transcripts were selected using the coding frame to identify quotations and extracts for use in this way.

# Conclusion

In this chapter we have provided an overview of the theoretical and methodological issues underpinning the examination of loneliness and isolation in later life. We have also outlined our argument for the appropriateness of a 'mixed-method' approach to the study of these concepts and described the two elements of our study design. However, as we argue in the next chapter, we also need to draw a wider focus and examine the 'non-pathological, non-problem' dimensions of social relationships in later life. In the following chapters we examine the empirical data concerning social participation, loneliness and isolation in later life.

# 3

# Social relations and everyday life

In the previous chapter we established the theoretical context for the book by considering different perspectives that may help our understanding of loneliness and isolation. In the next three chapters we examine the key empirical data describing older people's patterns of social engagement. Whilst we are looking throughout this book at the key issues of loneliness and isolation, we seek to embed this within a wider examination of the extent and type of social relationships engaged in by older people in their daily social lives. Where possible we look at common social patterns within the older population, but this group is by no means homogeneous. Indeed, it is now well accepted that issues of gender, age, ethnicity and class divide the older population, and that issues of generation differentiate the experience of 'old age' and later life. In taking this perspective, where possible we will examine cohort and generational related aspects of the social world of older people.

We start in this chapter by considering the range of activities and relationships within which older people are embedded by examining contacts with family and friends, participation in specific activities and the patterning of daily lives. Where available, we compare our findings with those from earlier research for there is much to be gained by locating contemporary patterns within an historical perspective. A wider view enables us to establish the continuities underpinning older people's engagement with the wider world and identify new and emerging patterns of social participation. We also seek, where possible, to draw comparisons with data from other countries as a way of further extending our understanding of the daily lives and social relationships of older people.

## Social participation and engagement

As we showed in Chapter 1 it is both well established and uncontroversial that the social environment is one of the key factors determining quality of life in old age as it is at earlier phases of the lifecycle (Bowling, 2005; Scharf et al., 2003). Quantitative research has consistently demonstrated a strong and positive relationship between social engagement in all forms, but especially participation within kin and wider social networks, and a higher quality of life. People of all ages routinely report that the social environment, especially social relationships with members of their family, is fundamental to notions of quality of life (Bowling, 1995). Typically older people report that seeing or being with family or friends and engaging in various forms of activities are the dimensions of life that bring 'happiness'. As one of Bowling's study participants states: 'The quality of my life now is my family' (Bowling, 2005: 91).

Recognition of the importance of the relationship between social engagement and 'quality of life' is not new. In the early 1960s, the largely American-based 'activity theorists' of ageing posited that the key to a good old age was the maintenance of kin and friendship-based relationships and participation and engagement with the wider social world via participation in formal activities such as church or volunteering. This resonates with the more contemporary ideas of Rowe and Kahn (1997) who suggest that a high level of social engagement is a key factor in achieving the goal of 'successful ageing'. Similar observations may be made about ideas such as 'healthy' ageing and active ageing: all place considerable emphasis upon the maintenance of social relationships and social participation as a key to achieving quality of life in old age. However, as Rowe and Kahn (1997) observe, the 'social support' needs to be of the 'right type at the right time' and there needs to be a goodness of fit – inappropriate or unwanted (or needed) support can be counter-productive and induce dependency instead of promoting independence. We can extend this observation into the realm of social participation more generally – in order to be effective, older people need to be engaged in social activities and relationships that are appropriate and meaningful for them. Identifying such activities, however, is challenging because of the diverse nature of the older population.

Whilst the prescriptive strictures and moral undertones of activity theory and successful aging remain subject to debate, the social environment continues to exert an important influence upon and context within which people experience old age. As social scientists we see that both conceptually and empirically the social context, of which social relationships form one vital part, exerts a critical influence upon the experience of later life. Social relationships can give 'meaning' to later life and provide the basis for giving and receiving support, both physical and emotional, to enable coping with life's vicissitudes regardless of age (Walker et al., 2005; Connidis, 2001 and 2005 and 2006).

Within the UK context, a key element of contemporary social policy thinking concerning the promotion of quality of life in later life relates to notions of social engagement and social inclusion (Office of the Deputy Prime Minister, 2006). This reflects a wider policy agenda concerned with enhancing 'social inclusion' and hence social cohesion across society, by strengthening social engagement and social ties, both formal and informal, which 'bind' individuals into society. This policy was initially articulated with specific reference to younger people and with a very heavy focus upon employment opportunities. However, the notion of 'social inclusion' has been translated across the generational divide to policy aimed specifically at older people.

A core objective for older people in the UK since 1945 has focused, in various guises, on the maintenance and enhancement of quality of life. Manipulation of the social environment by, for example, interventions to promote social engagement and combat loneliness and isolation may offer pathways to the achievement of this policy goal (Cattan et al., 2003 and 2005a and 2005b; Cattan and Ingold, 2003; Pinder and Hillier, 2001; Andrews et al., 2003; Stevens, 2001). Consequently there is a concern to promote social engagement amongst older people that is manifest in local, national and international policy-makers' interests in concepts such as 'social capital', 'social exclusion' and 'social inclusion'. However, the implicit objectives of such policies are subtly different from those emphasising social inclusion for younger age groups. With the younger age groups the concern has been to prevent social breakdown and the development of groups and subcultures detached from wider society, whilst for older people the focus is about promoting social ties as a way of ensuring the supply of 'informal care' – the majority of which is provided by family and friends (RIS MRC CFAS Resource Implications Study Group of the Medical Research Council Cognitive Function and Ageing Study, 1999).

We shall return to the detailed debates about the nature and definition of social exclusion in Chapter 5. In this chapter we detail the individual elements that fall within broad notions of exclusion and focus upon social participation and engagement. A recent report on social exclusion using data from the English Longitudinal Study of Ageing (ELSA) (Barnes et al., 2006) focused upon seven aspects of inclusion:

◆ Social relationships (contacts with family/friends)

◆ Cultural activities (going to the theatre/cinema)

◆ Civic activities (voting, volunteering and engagement in local interest groups)

◆ Access to basic services (shops, health services, etc.)

◆ Neighbourhood issues (feeling safe and secure)

◆ Financial products (banks)

◆ Material consumption (ability to afford household goods and holidays)

From this model, three dimensions – civic engagement, cultural engagement and social relationships – are strongly linked to the central concerns of this book and can be grouped together under the umbrella of 'social engagement'. Whilst we acknowledge the importance of material resources and other related factors these are not our prime focus. Social engagement is a broad and diverse concept with different subdivisions relating to notions such as social capital; social participation as measured by activity and contact rates; and social networks, which include notions of exchange relationships, intimate ties and differentiated roles (Scharf et al., 2004). Similarly, notions of social capital include ideas such as neighbourhood attachment, support networks, feelings of trust and reciprocity, local engagement, personal attachment to the area, feelings about safety, and proactivity in the social context. Within this book our focus is upon social relationships and participation, rather than more detailed network analysis.

However, by linking our quantitative and qualitative material we can examine both the extent of contacts and the nature and meaning of activities and relationships.

As we noted in the previous chapter, the predominant conceptualisation of exclusion in terms of social relationships in later life and the research literature more broadly has been in terms of investigating the 'pathological' end of the distribution with a specific concentration upon isolation and loneliness. There is a significant body of work describing and analysing these phenomena that largely reflects an approach to the investigation of social relationships in later life influenced by the study of 'social problems'. This goes with too ready an acceptance of the stereotype that the normal experience of old age is of social neglect, isolation and a reliance upon 'fragile' social networks. However, whilst isolation and loneliness are issues that afflict older people, they are neither universal nor restricted only or primarily to elders. Hence in this chapter we consider the wider social context and patterns of social relationships characterised by older people and locate these within notions of social engagement and social capital. In doing so we present a broader empirical characterisation of the extent of social engagement amongst older people. In presenting our empirical data we first examine relationships with family and friends and then consider participation in the wider social world and the degree to which older people are engaged within the spheres of inclusivity noted above. However, before we do this we describe the nature of our participants' personal understandings of old age and later life.

# The meaning of age: the backdrop to social relationships

We have described in some detail, both here and elsewhere (Bowling, 2005; Victor et al., 2005b), the quantitative characteristics of our participants in both components of our study. This enables us to present a statistical profile of our study participants and comment upon their representativeness (see Chapter 2). From this we can establish to what degree they are representative of the general population and evaluate demographic changes in the composition of the 'older population'. However, it does little to provide us with any insights into the 'worlds' of our participants and provide any insights on how they understood their worlds.

In our qualitative study, before introducing the specific questions concerned with their social world, participants were asked their views on age: Did their age effect the way they spent their time? Were they ever aware of their age? Did they feel it (age) was important? There was a widespread consensus amongst our participants on what constitutes the ageing process and how it affects people. Our participants saw ageing in terms of six major themes:

◆ General slowing down

◆ Risk assessments

◆ Deteriorating health

◆ Living for now

◆ Chronological age is immaterial

◆ Old is older than me

As we can see, two themes relate to deficits of deteriorating health and a general 'slowing down': one links to ideas about managing 'risk' – a way of combating age – whilst the others link to the meaning of age.

## 'Slowing down' with age

The ageing process was seen as a general slowing down. Things took longer to do and could not, and should not, be rushed. There was a need to 'plan', to ensure the successful accomplishment of required tasks. More time needed to be taken between tasks for recovery and relatively large tasks were split into smaller, manageable sections. Here we have a sense that, for our participants, ageing involved 'pacing' daily life and this would, of course, frame and contextualise any activities and relationships. As 'essential' tasks took longer to complete then, perhaps, we have a sense that there are fewer resources in terms of time and energy to spare for more social activities. We have a sense from our participants that the primary concern is with managing what are regarded as essential daily activities first and foremost. For example:

> I got the hoover out yesterday and did all the hoovering. I take my time you see. So this room will be done one day and then the bedroom will be hoovered and then it's the toilet that's got to be cleaned, and then the

spare room. But I do one a day. I pace myself because, you see, I get so tired. [210: 3: 14]

The pattern of your life changes, it slows down. As it should, I suppose, albeit I have to slowdown sometimes and take a deep breath. [305: 7: 32]

## Risk assessment

Risk assessment was applied not just to household chores but also to recreational activities such as gardening or participating in activities such as church. Our participants suggested that growing older was a 'risky' business, that there were more risks to be negotiated in daily life and that people needed to take more care physically as they got older. Some tasks were no longer considered appropriate, either by the individual themselves or, perhaps more importantly, by their relatives some of whom clearly saw old age as a 'risk management' activity. Decorating, manual work and heavy tasks around the house were considered carefully before our participants embarked on them.

[I see my] daughter, could be almost every day. But not necessarily. She comes in if I want anything like a light bulb put in or curtains changed round or something like that which I can't do myself. In fact I don't let myself do certain things which I used to do, in case I have a fall, or come off a ladder or something. Because I think if I do something then it will all come back on my daughter. [202: 4: 13]

This was particularly the case where ladders were involved. A number of people talked about no longer feeling safe up a ladder and, we can surmise, that the use of ladders was emblematic of the way that 'risks' of daily life were valuated and compensatory strategies developed in response to the challenges posed.

As I say, if I didn't get so tired doing things, I would tackle some of the decorating. In my garage I've got scaffolding and I used to erect the extension ladder and go right to the top of the gable of the house, but I can't now. I have to be careful when I get on the small pair of step ladders. There's nothing wrong but I have to be careful. [504: 7: 8]

This resulted in risk assessments being undertaken before people decided whether or not they would attempt tasks and also what the risks would be if they were to attempt the task and fail. Whilst these quotations link to the physical activities that older people were undertaking we can see how this easily translates into effecting their capacity for social engagement and their participation in social activities. There are clearly 'risk assessments' and 'cost-benefit' analyses being undertaken in respect of daily life, of which participation is just one element.

## Changes in health

Age was also seen in terms of an increase in health problems, or the emergence of health problems hitherto unknown. Rather than a feeling of deterioration, there was a feeling that problems had occurred as people got older that did not occur earlier on in their lives. Ageing was most definitely seen in terms of deteriorating health and our participants made a clear and conscious link between the two concepts.

> Well, generally speaking as you get older you have certain problems which you know you have, like eyesight, my hearing is beginning to go. I don't hear as well as I used to, and I haven't got as far as using a hearing aid yet which a lot of people have that are my age I think. [202: 9: 33]

Health problems, and particularly those effecting mobility, were seen as a nuisance or an irritation rather than anything more substantial. People with quite serious health problems still suggested that their health was generally OK and this reflects the consistent statistical discontinuity between the presence of 'objective' health problems and individuals' ratings of their own health, and the use of 'downward' comparisons and social positioning (Bowling, 2005).

> Q: Does your health or mobility affect what you do at all?
>
> A: I have a catheter now as a result of my prostate, which was benign fortunately. But ... er ... I learnt to live with it and I ... I can't walk as fast as I did, I mean that's just old age, I'm just slower in my movements. But I mean no, I ... I can't do as much as I used to or as much as I'd like to. I can't climb ladders as quick as I used to, that kind of thing that I used to do as a matter of course. You realise that as you get on. You're not capable of doing so many things so I do need help with some things. But so far life's been very good to me. [104: 7: 29]

Poor health, whilst perhaps not being a problem per se, was seen as getting in the way of people being able to lead the life they wanted to lead and as compromising independence and autonomy and clearly this would limit the potential for engagement. For our participants poor health and the consequent loss of their independence would be the worst thing that could possibly happen to them.

Q: So having your independence makes a huge difference then?

A: Yes. And the mobility and the health. The health comes first. Because if you don't have good health you can't do other things. [602: 6: 16]

One woman talked about her work in an 'old people's home'.

We always say God forbid that we're like this, let's hope someone puts us out of our misery before we get like this. But as you say, they don't know. They don't know they're incontinent and they make a mess and all that sort of thing. I know I wouldn't know about it but working with it. You know it might happen to you and that's frightening as you're getting older. [701: 8: 29]

Other examples were also given where friends had been 'put into' homes. One woman in particular expressed the desire to die, with dignity, in her own home.

My heart bleeds when I see nursing homes with old people sitting around waiting for God. In fact I've instructed my doctor that if I ever get like that ... I want to be left. I even asked my doctor if I can make a living will. I think people should be able to and he said to me it wouldn't be accepted. If you are in hospital they are there to preserve life. I don't want to end up in a nursing home. I said to [my son] when I go it'll be quick. But I don't worry about it. [603: 8: 7]

## 'Living for now'

Another way in which age was conceptualised was 'living for now'. A prevalent idea was that people lived in the present, or possibly in the past, but they were not living for the future as they had done when they were younger.

I've had dogs at various times, but when the last one had to be put down I decided it wasn't fair to start again. Well, not exactly fair, but that I probably wouldn't be able to cope with starting with another dog and all the problems involved with a new one in the house. [202: 2: 8]

You live in the here and now more don't you. You do unconsciously think of your mortality. This doesn't mean that you are worrying about whether this will be your last day but you don't think maybe in 10 years time I'll be doing this. [404: 9: 5]

One woman, in particular, talked about not feeling as if she was a part of the present day world, and not wanting to be a part of this world that she simply did not understand. With such a perspective it is unlikely that such participants will want to engage and participate in an external world that at best they find confusing and at worst frightening and disorientating.

I'm going back to before the war with all my time. I go back a lot. I'm content to keep to myself these days. I have nothing in common with what's going on in the world today. [603: 5: 25]

Another woman talked about being happier with what you have. She said that when she was younger she was always decorating her house, getting new furniture and so forth, but that now she has all she needs and is content to live with what she has got. There was a feeling of living for today rather than planning for the future. One man talked about this in terms of financial planning, gauging when it was the right time to break into their capital and start living off the money they had saved for their old age.

I'd like to see a bit more of the world before I go. But I think, a natural feeling of prudence there, I don't want to start yet dipping into reducing my capital, which is my intention eventually. As I say, I don't want to leave everything to the kids. But then that's one decision that [my wife] and I talk about, should we, while we are fit and well, be charging all over the place, and recognise the fact that there will come a time when we can't get around so easily. And we don't want to say, Oh I wish we'd done that then. [705: 8: 21]

He talked about moving from 'living for the future' to 'living for today'. With a changed, more present-centred focus, we might speculate that this does not encourage the development of new activities and relationships which require some 'future focus' to make such investments worthwhile.

## 'Chronological age is immaterial'

Within gerontology there is a significant body of work around the 'social construction' of 'old age' as a category (Jones, 2006; Powell,

2005 and 2006; Estes et al., 2003). All of our participants said that their chronological age was immaterial in the sense that they did not feel any different inside from the way that they did at the age of 30 or 40. These comments directly link to the ideas around the 'mask of ageing' (Featherstone and Hepworth, 1991; Ballard et al., 2005; Biggs, 1999) whereby the 'inner' young person is obscured by the mask of the older person.

> My age? You don't. When you get to my age, although the calendar shows that I'm 80 years old, my mind is the same as it was when I was 30 or 40 or 50 ... you don't feel that you're that old. [205: 7: 32]

One man suggested that although they may physically age, the real person inside does not age, they stay the same.

> The strange thing I find though, this question of being older, because the eyes that I look out on the world with I feel are the same eyes that I've always looked out with, and I don't feel that I'm old even though I know physically that I am 75. But I still feel strongly about, you know, world poverty, about injustice in the world, and I feel just as strongly about these sorts of social issues as I ever did. In a sense the real person doesn't change does it? [404: 9: 7]

He suggested that he felt just as strongly about all of the issues and passions he had cared about when he was younger, and that this part of him, his 'inner-self', had not changed, regardless of how his 'outer-self' may be changing. This is a paradigmatic illustration of ideas about continuity of identity across the life course.

## 'Old is older than me'

The final comment that our participants made about the issue of ageing was that 'old' was a category that referred to someone other than yourself. No matter how old you are, 'old' is someone other than you and our participants were very reluctant to adopt the 'spoilt identity' (Goffman, 1968) of the older person. This was a label that was negatively evaluated and was clearly one that should be resisted at almost all costs.

> I take an old lady shopping every Friday morning. I'm an old lady myself but she's older than me ... I do a bit of gardening. My husband's a gardener for the elderly. [503: 3: 1]

It is a category of otherness rather than one that you use to refer to yourself. This seems to be the case until people reach their 90s where the fact that they are 'old' seems to be an undeniable fact. As one woman pointed out:

And when you're older, I mean I'm not older, I'm the old, I'm jolly old. And I think it's more important to maintain your health because I'd hate to be incapacitated. To tell the truth, I'm feeling better than I have in years. [603: 4: 23]

Being 'old' is seen in terms of distinct categories. There are different levels of age: it is not categorised as a homogeneous group without internal dimensions of differentiation. One couple, who were both 83, talked about different levels of 'old age'. They suggested that warden-assisted flats, for example, can be a good thing, but that they themselves were not old enough to want (or need) one of those.

What my daughter wants is a place where you've got warden control. They're quite handy those you know. They have got a place down here, but I don't like the place down here. A friend of mine is down there and he went round the bend a bit. They can be good when you get older. But I'm not old enough yet. [208: 11: 6]

These later views demonstrate the use of 'positioning' (Jones, 2006) in that our participants were clearly locating themselves as not having the age status of the 'older' person and were identifying themselves as different from the group of people they thought of as old. Age here is being negotiated in a way that would probably not be true of gender amongst this group of participants. These views about old age and ageing provide a backdrop against which we can locate and interpret the empirical data about social relationships and participation.

## Family and friends

The changes in the nature and size of families in Britain over the past 60 years are well documented with reductions in family size and creation of 'blended families' via the impact of divorce and marriage breakdown in different generations (Harper and Kelly, 2003; Connidis, 2005; Harper, 2006). Indeed, this constitutes one of the major secular trends that provide a context within which we present our analysis of social relationships. The creation of new relationship trajectories such as 'serial monogamy' and the development of civil partnerships show that the 'family' continues to be a dynamic and constantly changing, highly flexible unit of social organisation. However, we must be cautious in seeing family disruption and 'breakdown' as being a 'new' social phenomenon. There have always been families consisting of single parents and blended families based upon re-marriage and 'step' relationships. What marks out the current situation is the reason for family disruption, mainly divorce and relationship breakdown rather than death as in previous generations, together with more prevalent experience of complex family organisational frameworks.

Whilst our study did not set out to establish the social and family structure of participants we can present an overview of family ties for contemporary older people. This complements the more locally based studies of Phillipson et al. (2001) and offers a framework for interpreting our empirical material, both quantitative and qualitative. It also offers an opportunity to present data on secular trends and provides the context within which to contextualise family-based relationships and levels of contact. In this section we are concerned with documenting the availability of kin relationships prior to examining levels of contact and engagement and the context and meaning attached to such contacts.

The majority of our participants (61 per cent) in the quantitative study were married, with one per cent cohabiting. As with other social surveys women are less likely to be married than men – 47 per cent compared with 73 per cent, and the percentage classified as widowed increases with age from 18 per cent at aged 65–74 to 43 per cent at ages 85 years and over. However, there was little variation between ages and gender in terms of the percentages classified as divorced, separated and single (never married). The decline of the female spinster group so visible in the surveys of Sheldon (1948), Shanas et al. (1968) and Hunt (1978) is evident from examination of Table 2.3 in the previous chapter where 11–15 per cent of their samples were single women compared with about five per cent of our participants.

## Widowhood

Undoubtedly the experience of bereavement is especially disruptive in that, for many of us, the relationship with our spouse or partner is the axis upon which our social world is founded. As we shall discuss further in the next two chapters, widowhood is associated with isolation, exclusion and loneliness. Overall 27 per cent of our survey participants were widowed. Of these, seven per cent had been bereaved within one year of the survey, 13 per cent for between one and three years and two-thirds (66 per cent) for over five years. The impact of such an event, especially after marriages of considerable longevity is evident in the words of one of our participants.

Q: And how long were you married for?

A: Almost 56 years. Just two months short. We were married on 27th December 1944 and my husband died on 30th October last year. So Christmas we would have been married for 56 years. He was everything you could ever want in a husband. That's why I miss him so much you see. But still, you can't have it forever. [301: 1: 33]

This reflects the importance of the spouse relationship across the life course. Data from the English Longitudinal Study of Ageing report that, for those aged 50 years and over, at least 75 per cent described their relationship with their spouse as 'very close' (Barnes et al., 2006). Although the majority of widows and widowers in our survey, 66 per cent, had been widowed for five years or longer, it is easy to underestimate the impact of bereavement when it is a much less recent event. As these participants indicated, although a considerable number of years may have passed, the impact of the event can still be very immediate and very raw.

You see after my husband died everyone said how marvellous I was, I kept up because I had three girls at home. It was after they left home. Then I was really on my own and it really hit me. 23 years ago this November John died. Very sudden it was, very very sudden. I was 46. [405: 4: 12]

## Children

In the survey most older people, 87 per cent, had living children. This is very similar to the data reported by Townsend (1957), Bond and Carstairs (1982) and (Wenger, 1984) and in line with the 86 per cent of those aged 50 years and over with children reported by the English Longitudinal Study of Ageing (Barnes et al., 2006). Whilst the percentage of older people with children is largely stable, the number of children per family has undoubtedly reduced over the timeframe covered in these studies, although there are no directly comparable data available from studies to illustrate this. However, this may not be true for future generations of elders where rates of childlessness amongst some cohorts are approximately 20 per cent. With the effects of mortality this is likely to increase (Evandrou and Falkingham, 2000; Harper, 2006). For those older people who have children, parents and children are experiencing very much longer relationships than in the past (because of increased longevity) and these relationships are as 'independent adults' rather than the parent–child dependent relationship characteristic of previous generations.

The classic post-war studies of specific communities such as London, Swansea and Wolverhampton demonstrated the extensive co-residence of older people and their adult children. However, what is more difficult to determine is the degree to which this was 'voluntary' or was a reflection of a very acute post-Second World War housing crisis and poverty. We can illustrate this by reference to the example of Swansea. In the initial survey by Rosser and Harris (1965) in 1960, 16 per cent of participants lived in 'three-generational' households. The resurvey of Swansea in 2002 revealed that two per cent now lived in this form of household (Charles et al., 2003). They also report that, in 1960, 20 per cent of families lived in extended households consisting of parents and their married children. The extent of social change in terms of co-residence across generations is that in the 2002 re-survey only five households were so categorised (Charles et al., 2003). This is one feature of contemporary society that has changed dramatically but what is more contentious is what this 'means' socially. How is this change understood between the differing generations involved? What impact will this change have upon inter-generational relationships? In addition, changes in longevity mean that for contemporary cohorts of elders they are much more likely to be members of three-, four- or even five-generation families but very much less likely to reside within multiple generation households.

With this data about domestic co-residence in mind, how spatially close are older people to their children nowadays? Has co-residence been replaced by living in the same areas or neighbourhoods? In our survey almost two-thirds, 61 per cent of those with children, lived within five miles of them whilst 16 per cent lived over 50 miles away and two per cent lived abroad (Table 3.1). These data resonate with

**Table 3.1** Geographical proximity of children and siblings (per cent)[1]

|  | Children | Sibling |
|---|---|---|
| Same house/within 1 mile | 33 | 14 |
| 1–5 miles | 29 | 22 |
| 6–15 miles | 13 | 15 |
| 16–50 miles | 7 | 14 |
| 50+ miles | 16 | 30 |
| Abroad | 2 | 5 |
| Total | 100 | 100 |
| (Number) | (867) | (698) |

[1] Question relates to geographically closest child/sibling.

those of Phillipson et al. (2001b) and, perhaps surprisingly, show considerable similarity with more historical data. Phillipson and colleagues (Phillipson et al., 1998) report that three studies (Abrams, 1978; Rosser and Harris, 1965; Young and Willmott, 1957) from the 1950s to the early 1970s report that between 80–64 per cent of older people had children living within five miles of their residence.

So we can see that there is some continuity over time – in the past not everyone's children lived next door in a cosy 'Coronation Street' world. In a recent analysis Grundy and Shelton (2001) showed that 76 per cent of older people had children living within one mile of them in 1953 compared with 23 per cent in 2000. This reflects the change over the past 60 years in household living arrangements that we have already reported, but suggests that although parents and children have established separate residences these are generally within a reasonably close geographical distance with only a third of our survey participants living over five miles away from their nearest child. Of course what we cannot glean from this is who moved away from whom. However, we should also note that for 13 per cent of our sample their nearest living child was resident at least 50 miles away and 1.5 per cent lived abroad. Few surveys undertaken in the 1960s included either of these categories in their response set. Hence we can draw inferences from the changing nature and assumptions about family relationships by the questions asked by social surveys of older people before even moving on to the analysis of the answers! Our questions and response categories provide useful insights into contemporary social concerns and ideologies.

However, we should be cautious of generalising from locality-based studies since they often relate to very specific and highly localised geographical communities. We also need to take the spatial and temporal dimension into account when interpreting historical data. Rosser and Harris (1965) report that their data for the proximity of adult children to parents in Swansea is very similar to that of Young and Willmott (1957) in Bethnal Green – about 70 per cent living in the same 'locality'. However, at the time of these two studies, Swansea had an area of 41 square miles and Bethnal Green 1.5 so the meaning and area covered by the term 'locality' is clearly very different in the two studies. Having posed this caveat we should not underplay the influence that spatial distance can have upon the link between older people and their adult children. As some of our participants explained:

Q: So how often do you see your daughter then?

A: Erm well, when she lived here I used to see her every week ... I see them about once a month. As I say I used to see her every week. But now it's once a month. [503: 3: 14]

... my daughter that's in Jersey, I see her three to four times a year, she has to come over. The one in Scotland I saw at Easter time, and that's the first time for three or four years because they were abroad. And the one in Italy I used to see every week you see, once or twice a week. So suddenly the bottom fell out of my world. But there you are, it can't be helped. I can't stand in the way of my children. [703: 1: 45]

This illustrates the mediating effect that geographical distance can have and how an older person's social web can be influenced by external forces such as adult children moving to find employment. However, we must also be wary of inferring that proximity invariably results in high levels of contact.

Q: What about your family then, how often do you see them?

A: Not very often, they've got their own families, they've got their own families. I mean I've got a daughter lives within 10 minutes ... I sometimes see her when she takes her daughter to school, that's about the only time I do see her, when she goes by taking the young uns to school. I never see me son. [702: 6: 20–24]

## Siblings

Almost three quarters, 70 per cent, of our survey participants had siblings, again not dissimilar to previous research such as the 78 per cent reported by Bond and Carstairs (1982) and these showed a pattern of more geographical dispersion with 37 per cent living within five miles and 30 per cent living over 50 miles away. Hence there seems to be greater spatial distance between siblings rather than children and their parents although, again, our cross-sectional survey does not enable us to comment upon either the recency (or otherwise) of this arrangement or which of the siblings moved! However, we should not underestimate either the importance of siblings in the social lives of older people or the importance of contact between siblings. Perhaps surprisingly this has often been underplayed in previous research where the emphasis was very much upon the importance of children and grandchildren.

> I've got two brothers and I did have two sisters but sadly I lost my eldest sister last year, she died. But I've got a sister in [name of town] which is local. We always kept in touch, we always visited. [405: 2: 3]
>
> My sister takes up a lot of my time and of course my grandchildren down in Canterbury ... I've got a brother in Australia ... I've got a sister who lives in Harrow on the Weald ... And then I have another sister who lives in Derbyshire ... [503: 5: 1]

This participant's response nicely illustrates the dispersed but still highly meaningful and important relationships that siblings can have across the life course and that transcend geographical barriers. There is considerable scope for studying sibling relationships across the life course and in old age. We also need to note that for future cohorts of elders there will be fewer who will bring the experience of direct first degree kin relatives to old age but many more who will grow old in the company of their step and half siblings. So for future cohorts there may (or may not) be subtle changes in the nature of sibling relationships in later life. We feel that there is an extensive research agenda to be developed looking at continuities and discontinuities of sibling relationships across the life course and the emerging and evolving nature of sibling bonds (Cicirelli, 1995; Connidis, 2001).

Geography and environment are both clearly important but family and friendship-based relationships do not equate simply to a simple distance-related algorithm. Proximity does not necessarily engender intimacy and vice versa. For 40 per cent of the survey participants the family member they felt closest too was not geographically close. Similarly 21 per cent reported that the friend they felt closest to was not local to them. Hence disentangling the link between geographical proximity, the time and ease with which the distance can be covered, the recency of the geographical separation, the quality of the relationship and degree of direct physical contact is complex. This paradox of having close relationships with people with whom we are separated by time or distance has led to the development of the concept of intimacy at a distance. This is a world away from the communities described by Townsend (1957), Young and Willmott (1957) and Rosser and Harris (1965) where intimate social relationships were confined to a relatively small geographical area, although as these authors restricted their attention to defined localities it is unclear if there were more distant and meaningful relationships that demonstrated 'intimacy at a distance'.

However, we also need to recognise that some older people have limited family ties. Whilst this is the minority experience we need to remember that there are individuals without the family links described above. As one unmarried participant reported:

> . . . they're pretty remote, I originally had four first cousins, two on my father's side who were more than ten years older than me, and two on my mother's side who are more than ten years younger than me, so I never really had anything very much to do with my first cousins. So now I have to say that my next of kin is the son of one of the older ones who is a second cousin. But he lives in Shropshire. I have seen him once this year because he came to visit me, when I had my hip operation. Normally if I get a phone call during the year then I'm lucky and I get a Christmas card. We're not close. [207: 3: 25–32].

## Contact with family, friends and neighbours

Having framed the continuities and changes in the availability and proximity of family and kin we now consider, empirically, the levels of contact between older people and their family, friends and neighbours.

In the measurement of social contacts, the inclusion and exclusion of particular kin relationships and wider social relationships such as friends and neighbours has been specific to different studies and researchers. The quality of interactions was rarely evaluated and assumptions were clearly made about the importance of certain relationships, such as the husband-wife and mother-daughter relationships, over other relationships, even though at the time the empirical evidence for these judgements was lacking. A contextual feature of these early studies was the focus on physical contact encapsulated in the question 'How often do you see X?' Other methods of contact, increasingly prevalent in the twenty-first century, such as phone conversations or internet communication via email or on-line conversations were not included (for obvious reasons) in the earlier studies. But there appears to be a time lag in the inclusion of such technologically induced social change in later studies measuring social isolation. It is not until the national study reported by Hunt (1978) that the telephone was asked about as a method of promoting and maintaining social relationships rather than as a means of 'emergency' contact. But from a common-sense perspective counting the number of social contacts, however you define contact, probably provides an objective measure of social contact as long as the quality of relationships, duration of relationships and interaction and the weighting of significant relationships is not seen as an essential feature of social isolation. Hence in our study we asked participants to report their frequency of contact with family, friends and relatives via a variety of media using questions derived from the national General Household Survey. This has enabled us to consider the generalisability of our findings and to address cross-generational levels of engagement. In addition, as we saw in Chapter 1, these questions are broadly typical of those used in other social surveys of older people in Britain. However, as our questions collect responses in terms of categories or broad levels of contacts rather than absolute numbers, this limits the precision of any calculated 'social isolation' index composed solely from these variables. We discuss the definition and calculation of our measures of isolation and exclusion further in Chapter 5.

Levels of direct contact between older people and their family and friends remains high. Table 3.2 indicates that 22 per cent of those aged 65 years and over are in direct phone contact with their family daily, 13 per cent are in direct daily contact and 62 per cent see relatives at least once a week.

**Table 3.2** Contact with family, friends and neighbours (per cent)[1]

|  | Speak to relatives on phone | See relatives | Speak to friends on phone | See friends | Speak to neighbours | Send/ receive letters | Send/ receive emails |
|---|---|---|---|---|---|---|---|
| Every day | 22 | 13 | 11 | 15 | 36 | 1 | 0 |
| 5–6 days per week | 5 | 6 | 3 | 5 | 8 | 0 | 1 |
| 3 or 4 days a week | 15 | 13 | 16 | 17 | 18 | 1 | 3 |
| Once or twice a week | 36 | 30 | 34 | 34 | 27 | 6 | 2 |
| Once or twice a month | 10 | 20 | 18 | 14 | 6 | 19 | 2 |
| Once every couple of months | 3 | 9 | 4 | 5 | 3 | 17 | 2 |
| Once or twice a year | 2 | 7 | 6 | 5 | 1 | 33 | 2 |
| Not in last year | 3 | 3 | 7 | 4 | 1 | 23 | 90 |
| (Number) | (994) | (993) | (992) | (992) | (994) | (994) | (993) |
| Total | 100 | 100 | 100 | 100 | 100 | 100 | 100 |

[1] Totals may not sum to 100% because of rounding

This mixed portfolio of forms of contact is illustrated by our participants who commented thus:

My daughter rang me just before you came. She rings from Italy once or twice a week, you know, just to keep in touch. Tom, that's the grandson in London, rings about the same number of times, and he comes down about once a month or so. [905: 3: 34–6]

Oh yes we phone up nearly every day, my phone bill is quite heavy but I don't mind that, I'm not spending money on other things. And my sister in Norwich I talk to her regularly once or twice a week, I'm going to see her next Tuesday. I phone her every Sunday, well usually on a Sunday and we'll talk for over an hour. Or she'll phone me, same with my other sister, the same with the family. I mean I get a phone call every day from one member of the family. I mean that my granddaughter, I was telling my son the other day, she's teaching in Sevenoaks, she phones me up every week, she phoned me up last night, she's only 23. And she never misses. So every day there's somebody on the phone, or a friend. [301: 2: 41–50]

The levels of contact are consistent with those reported in other contemporary surveys involving older people such as the General Household Survey (GHS) which reported that 79 per cent of those aged 65 and over saw their relatives or friends (no distinction in the published tables is drawn between these two groups) weekly and this level of contact has remained roughly stable since 1980 when the GHS first introduced these social contact questions for older people (Victor, 2005). These high levels of contact with friends support the work of Jerrome and Wenger (1999) who argued for the importance of friendship networks in promoting 'quality of life' in old age.

One key element of social cohesion and feelings of community are notions of the role and importance of neighbours and neighbourliness (Bernard et al., 2001; Phillipson et al., 1999) and the link to the local neighbourhood (Joong-Hwan, 2003). Contact with neighbours is most frequently reported – with 88 per cent of older people reporting speaking to neighbours weekly and 29 per cent speaking to them daily. These levels of contact with neighbours are slightly higher than the 78 per cent reported by the 2000 GHS and again the levels recorded by the GHS have remained roughly stable over the past two decades. Whilst these data record the degree of contact between older people and their family and friends and neighbours we can only speculate that the nature and meaning of contacts with neighbours for many older people is rather different from contacts with family or friends. Indeed, the semantic differences between friends and neighbours is not often clear. Typically neighbours were described thus and were a category distinct from friends but not unimportant.

Finally, the notion of 'people we know' who were neither friends, relatives or neighbours was a recurrent theme as this exchange illustrates:

Q: And do you have any friends in this area?

A: People we know. Just people we know, that's all.

Q: So do you know some of the neighbours then?

A: Yes, to talk to, but ... I wouldn't class them as friends, would you?, just people we know. I mean down there we made some very good friends. Down there. But here, no. [403: 5: 45]

How such relationships are categorised when participants were asked in the quantitative element of the study about contact with neighbours/

friends is of interest. Researchers devise questions that require survey participants to evaluate social relationships according to predefined categories, predominantly family, friends and neighbours. However, these two quotes suggest that these categories are not always clear cut, that there are intermediate categories and that the term 'neighbour' carries connotations of proximity and co-residence that is not always required of friends (see Phillipson et al., 1999).

However, as the qualitative element of our study illustrates, neighbours can be very important as this comment demonstrates:

> ... well and the neighbours, I don't, the neighbours opposite, they're lovely. I see quite a bit of them. But we don't live in each other's houses if you know what I mean. I saw her this morning and had a long chat and we always tell each other when we're going away so that we can keep an eye on each other's properties and so on. Erm, we have the occasional evening out together, you know, but the other neighbours I'm friendly with, when we meet we chat, but not to go into their houses. [303: 26–31]

Friends are also important. In the English Longitudinal Study of Ageing, 91 per cent of those aged 50 years and over reported that they 'had friends'. Although the percentages declined with age, 83 per cent of those aged 80 years and over reported that they had friends (Barnes et al., 2006). In our study 15 per cent of participants saw friends daily and 11 per cent talked with them on the phone daily and almost two-thirds talked with friends on the phone at least weekly and a similar percentage, 71 per cent, saw their friends at least weekly (Table 3.2). In the English Longitudinal Study of Ageing, 59 per cent of participants aged 50 and over saw friends weekly and 58 per cent talked to them on the phone weekly, compared with 71 per cent and 64 per cent respectively in our study. Visiting and being visited by friends was perceived as important in daily life and particularly a part of having a good quality of life.

> If I hadn't got good friends the days would drag. I mean there is a limit to the things you can do in a house aren't there? [302: 5: 28]

However, a key theme in many of our qualitative interviews was the diminishing pool of long-established friends as the cumulative effects of frailty and mortality reduced friendship networks with little opportunity to renew them. Similar observations were reported by the participants in Phillipson et al.'s (1999) study.

> ... that is a problem, because a lot of friends that we've got are beginning to disappear. And I suppose a big problem is when you get a bit older and then most of your friends have died. [201: 3: 44]

> When you get to my age you don't make lasting friends because you haven't got that long ... we had loads of friends. The last one died at 87 of throat cancer last year. They were my age group. Every year there would be a Christmas card less to send as they died each year. [603: 6: 34]

## Trends in social contacts

A key question in our project was the degree to which there have (or have not) been changes in the levels of social contact between older people and their family, friends and neighbours and indeed the wider social world. How do the patterns of social contact noted earlier mesh with those reported by previous surveys? It is problematic to establish unambiguously because of the differing way this topic has been investigated by previous researchers. Even two recent surveys such as ours and the English Longitudinal Study of Ageing show differences in how questions are asked – they enquired separately about contacts with children and other relatives and we did not; they did not use a 'daily' response category but we did. This illustrates the point that different surveys use different question wording and have specific issues that they wish to address in response to the specific socio-spatial context within which they are undertaken. We can illustrate this point further by using the example of the survey undertaken by Hunt (1978). She examines contact between older people and their families and friends in great detail. In particular, she draws a distinction between, for example, visits made to or received from relatives but not always distinguishing the differing relationships of family and friends. Unfortunately it is not possible from her published work to determine overall levels of contact without re-analysis of the data. Similarly, Rosser and Harris (1965) and Young and Willmott (1957) present details about contact between older people and their married sons and daughters but do not report overall levels of contact nor any details of contact with unmarried children or more distant relatives. Surveys also vary in the reference reporting periods or the periods over which contacts are enumerated. Additionally there is a tradition in established surveys to focus upon direct social contacts rather than other forms of engagement.

One source which enables us to develop an historical perspective on social contacts in later life and which demonstrates reasonable consistency of question wording, relationships enquired about and response categories is the General Household Survey. This dataset has the merit of using fairly consistent question format and response categories. Using this source as we suggest earlier, there has been very little change since 1980 in levels of social interaction between older people and family, friends and neighbours although we cannot comment upon how the quality or meaning of such relationships may have changed over time. Comparison of our data with those from Tunstall might hint at a slight increase in contacts. Tunstall (1966) reports that 25 per cent of his sample saw relatives three or more times a week and 27 per cent friends – in our survey 32 per cent saw relatives three times or more a week and 37 per cent saw friends. If we factor in telephone contact levels of overall contact may be higher than previously reported. Whilst that could be described as an over-optimistic statement of our data, it certainly does not suggest a pattern of decline and may reflect increased rates of social activity by contemporary cohorts of older people, especially with friends, reflecting their greater level of (relative) affluence and health and increased forms of contact via phone and email compared with their 1960s equivalents.

Whilst the overall pattern of older people's contacts with family, friends and neighbours may be characterised as broadly stable there have been changes in the nature of these contacts as noted above. One very clear difference is in the nature of social engagements. Since Sheldon's (1948) study, the nature of social interaction has changed radically. In the immediate post-Second World War period the majority of social interactions were direct 'face-to-face' interchanges, with letters forming the most common manifestation of non-contact social relations. For example, Townsend (1957) only asked about direct contacts and Hunt (1978) was concerned with the distinctions of visits and visiting. None of the surveys of this period asked about telephone-based contact (Shanas et al., 1968; Hunt, 1978; Bond and Carstairs, 1982). The growth of communications technologies, initially telephones but now email and other IT-based methods, has expanded the arenas in which social relationships can be fostered.

In the 1970s Hunt (1978) reported that only 45 per cent of her sample had a telephone. At the beginning of the twenty-first century, at the time of our fieldwork, fixed-line phone ownership was virtually 100 per cent and one-third of older people had a mobile phone. Clearly the telephone has become an increasingly important aspect of older people's contact with their family and friends. Table 3.2 shows that 78 per cent of older people talked at least weekly to relatives on the phone and 64 per cent to their friends. As yet we can only speculate as to the potential for IT-led communication methods for enmeshing older people within family and friendship networks.

The following interview extract nicely illustrates a combination of themes: the adoption of new technology by older people, often at the behest of younger relatives for surveillance reasons but which can be used very positively to promote communication and relationships within the family and the wider community.

> They brought me this mobile so they could check on me. I was walking the dog Monday morning and ... click, click, click. I thought what the Dickens is that. And then I realised it were that thing going off. Somebody on the other end of the line says 'Good morning granddad'. I said 'Good morning'. He said 'I expect you're just walking in the woods?', I says 'Yes'. 'What's the weather like?', I says 'Very, very nice'. He says 'Now don't walk too far. Just be careful what you're doing.' I says, 'What's going off here.' I says, 'What're you doing?' He says, 'I'm just going to school', he says 'but I thought I'd ring you to make sure you were alright before I went.' And he's 13! So they think a bit of their Granddad (laughs). Aye it were grand. I have fun with them. They're very caring people. I don't know how some of these people cope, you keep reading about them in the paper, you know, they haven't got anybody. I don't know. [402: 6: 30]

New media such as email and webcasting offer the potential for older people to maintain relationships and engage in social interaction. They are an obvious method for maintaining 'intimacy at a distance' and a way of overcoming the barriers to communication posed by frailty and spatial separation as well as offering potential opportunities for surveillance, monitoring and intervention or service provision. However, they do require access to appropriate technology, the expertise to use the equipment and the inclination to communicate via such remote links. In our survey 12 per cent of participants were in email contact with family or friends annually, with six per cent reporting this happened on an at least weekly basis. This seems likely to expand considerably over future decades but our study was too early to capture the activities of the emerging 'silver surfers'.

## Social support

Whilst the approach in our project was to look at social relationships in 'the round' we cannot exclude the 'support' dimension of social relationships. In terms of practical support or exchange relationships over 90 per cent of our participants reported that there was someone they could ask for a lift in an emergency, who would provide help if they were in bed or give help at home or provide support in a personal crisis (Table 3.3). Indeed 78 per cent reported that there was someone they could ask for help if they had a financial crisis. As we can see in Table 3.3, the bedrock of the support network that older people would turn to in the event of these varying threats and crises are rooted within the family, although the importance of friendships in providing support should not be underestimated. As one participant succinctly observed 'we get support from our friends' [201: 44].

The importance of neighbours with practical instrumental tasks and activities is also important and echoes the work of Phillipson et al.

**Table 3.3** If you needed help with specific problems (per cent)[1]

|  | Needed a lift | Ill in bed | Financial difficulties | Help with daily chores |
|---|---|---|---|---|
| Help available (%) | 91 | 96 | 78 | 91 |
| *Provided by (%)* |  |  |  |  |
| Spouse/partner | 33 | 52 | 33 | 39 |
| Relative | 58 | 62 | 79 | 55 |
| Friends | 45 | 29 | 17 | 33 |
| Neighbours | 48 | 32 | 4 | 38 |
| Other | 4 | 4 | 0 | 3 |
| Prefer not to ask for help | 1 | 1 | 8 | 1 |

[1] Multiple response permitted

(2001). Neighbours can also be a link with the immediate family and help in an emergency.

> A: I've got two good neighbours either side. If they haven't seen me about they want to know why, so that's nice.
>
> Q: So have you got people that you could ask for help if you needed something or wanted to talk to someone?
>
> A: Yeah, well next door, I can ring them, or the other side. Well I always see the other side, she gets my tea from Sainsburys every week. I've only got to ring. And if they (family) can't get me on the phone they ring next door and they come round and see what's happened. [105: 5: 1–5]

> When my sister-in-law fell in the garden and I was away the son heard something and looked out and he knew my number and phoned me and then he took her to the accident treatment centre so I met up with them there. [504: 3: 35–7]

It is all too easy to see older people as recipients of support from their social network without also remembering that they are also providers of support to others. Whilst we cannot comment upon the detail, our data show that in addition to being recipients of support, our older people were also providers of support as this interview extract illustrates:

> I dread the phone ringing at times, now that is not true. Because I'm in reasonably good health and I drive I tend to fill in the gaps let's say it is much as my youngest son is the police officer and he works shifts. My daughter-in-law works part-time at Marks & Spencer's and that usually works out quite well but when my son is on late shift he can't pick the children up from school, so I go and pick them up from school and stay there until their mother gets home from work. These are the ones that are in Colchester. And then if my son is in court on a case and he realises he is not going to get away in time I get an urgent phone call can you go and pick the boys up, you know. That sort of thing, and I also have them quite a lot in school holiday time. [305: 4: 10–14]

Older people also helped neighbours as well as receiving help from them as this illustrates:

> Q: So do you know the neighbours quite well then if you've lived here for 30 years?
>
> A: Yes. Well, on a nodding acquaintance. The lady next door's got

multiple sclerosis and I've got the key to her flat and I do one or two
things for her. [505: 1: 31–4]

Hence older people play both roles within their support networks, the
balance of caring activities presumably varying over the life course.

In terms of 'intimate or confiding' relationships, which have long
been associated with both good quality of life and positive mental
health, 60 per cent of our participants reported that they had at least
one relative and 70 per cent at least one friend living nearby that they
felt 'close' to. Furthermore, 99 per cent of participants felt that there
was someone they could turn to who would provide comfort and
support in times of personal crisis. Examples of these forms of support
include:

I mean my daughter, me oldest daughter, I've got a wonderful relationship with her, we have got a great relationship. [406: 5: 45–6]

Oh yes. One that was here yesterday, great friend. I only have to pick up
the phone and she'd be here. Yeah. I mean it was the same when her
husband died. She picked up the phone and we were there. It's just, I
mean they'd been great friends for years. And I think you could, some of
the people that still live in the village, you know the older people, you
could go and say. You know I've got a problem can you help me, and
they will. I don't think you'd have any problems here not getting help if
you needed it. [701: 6: 15–21]

## Participation in the wider social world

Our analysis so far has focused upon the relationships and contacts
between older people and their family and friends. How active and
engaged are older people in the wider social world and their
neighbourhood?

### The neighbourhood and social relationships

Older age, like other phases of the life course, is enacted within a spatial
as well as social framework. Indeed, the early community-based studies
of Bethnal Green, Swansea and Dagenham were very aware of the
importance of the spatial and neighbourhood environment in facilitating and contextualising relationships. This has been re-emphasised
by the recent work of Scharf and colleagues (2004) and Peace et al.

(2005). The immediate neighbourhood is of particular importance to the well-being and quality of life of older people (Bowling, 2006). Whilst there has been much focus on the importance of maintaining older people at 'home' this has often been interpreted as the narrow confines of the built dwelling or house rather than the wider environment of neighbourhood or locality. Yet place is clearly important in providing the spatial context within which old age (and other phases of the life course) is established (Berkman et al., 2000; Berkman and Glass, 2000). The locality can shape social experience but remained until recently a comparatively neglected aspect of the gerontological research (Peace et al., 2005; Phillipson, 2007; Scharf et al., 2007). Furthermore, Bowling (2005) has argued that place or neighbourhood is an under-appreciated dimension of social capital as broadly defined. Certainly the inclusion of an explicit dimension of 'neighbourhood' in the current model of social exclusion demonstrates that the importance of place is now recognised within a broader policy context.

How do older people feel about where they live? Bowling (2005) has discussed this extensively in her book on quality of life and elsewhere (Bowling and Stafford, 2007). However, some of the key findings merit reiteration for they both re-emphasise the importance of place but also serve to combat some of the stereotypes about older people. In the broadest sense social capital is concerned with shared values, social ties, a sense of belonging and feelings of association that combine to increase the available social resources of individuals. The majority of older people in our survey, 92 per cent, enjoyed living in their area, although only a third felt that their locality or neighbourhood was above average in terms of facilities for those aged 65 years and over. Much is made of the vulnerability felt by older people in terms of crime and when out walking. Just under a quarter, 24 per cent, of participants felt that crime was a big or fairly big problem in their area, 88 per cent felt safe whilst walking alone during the day and 35 per cent felt safe walking alone at night. This feeling of 'safety' whilst walking, especially in the day, is somewhat higher than in the English Longitudinal Study of Ageing. However, it is an important factor as 'fear' – of crime or other dangers, whether real or imagined – is a major barrier to participating in the wider social world. Hence overall our participants did not feel especially threatened by the environment in which they lived. This is reflected in the observation that only two per cent of

participants stated that they did not know people in their neighbourhood – 50 per cent reported that they knew many or most of the people
in their neighbourhood and 72 per cent that they trusted the people in
their neighbourhood. So at a general population level for older people
the neighbourhood is one of familiarity where they know and trust the
majority of residents. However, our data represent a 'national overview' and as Phillipson et al. (2001) and Scharf et al. (2007) note there
are pockets, predominantly in inner-city areas, where the experience of
older people in terms of their immediate environment is less favour-
ably evaluated. Furthermore, as the study by Jakobsson and Hallberg
(2005) indicates, fear of crime is associated with loneliness.

## Civic and cultural activities

In reporting social participation we are interested in older people's
involvement with civic and cultural activities since they link with the
model of social exclusion developed by Scharf et al. (2007). Overall 24
per cent of participants had taken part in one (or more) of the range of
activities listed in Table 3.4 in the previous month and seven per cent
had undertaken none of them. Table 3.4 reports participation in the

**Table 3.4** Participation in activities (% participating in various activities)

| | |
|---|---|
| **Civic activities** | |
| Voted in last election | 81 |
| Undertaken voluntary work[1] | 16 |
| Used library[1] | 40 |
| Attended church/mosque etc[1] | 29 |
| Attended local organisation[1] | 42 |
| Attended educational/evening class[1] | 7 |
| **Cultural activities** | |
| Gone to cinema, theatre[1] | 29 |
| **Physical activities** | |
| Gone for a walk[1] | 68 |
| Played sport, gone swimming, etc. | 20 |
| Gardening[1] | 59 |
| Helping activities | |
| Babysitting/childminding[1] | 24 |
| Looked after someone who was ill/frail[1] | 17 |

[1] In the previous month

formal civic fabric of society through to more leisure-based activities, although the degree of social interaction encompassed by, for example, going for a walk or gardening is unclear. Nevertheless it is an indication that individuals are part of an external world and that life's activities are not restricted entirely to the confines of the built home. We had more limited data on cultural activities – 29 per cent of participants had been to the theatre or cinema in the previous month. The most frequently reported activities were walking (68 per cent) and gardening (59 per cent). Involvement in a sporting activity such as swimming was reported by 29 per cent of survey participants.

Within the current debate about social exclusion, participation in 'civic society', as illustrated by voting, participating in local democracy and participation in faith or community groups, is viewed as problematic for young or mid-life adults. The topic is rarely extended to older people, although as Table 3.4 indicates older people do contribute to the civic life of their communities by either involvement or use of organisations and facilities. Some 80 per cent of survey participants had voted in the last election; this is very similar to the 80 per cent reported for those aged 50 plus in the English Longitudinal Study of Ageing (Barnes et al., 2006). Some 42 per cent of participants were attending a local club or organisation. These organisations were many and varied but their importance for members, who had often been involved for many years, is typified by the following:

I have another identity because my hobby is magic and I have a stage name and in that sphere that's how I'm known by everybody. I'm in a society that meets weekly. I was president for 34 years. The last 30 consecutive. And they made me president emeritus at the end of it all. So that is a main interest in life and I produce a magazine every month for them and that's how I spend quite a bit of my time. [504: 3: 35–7].

Overall 16 per cent were involved in voluntary work. Writing from a North American perspective Martinson and Minkler (2006) note how civic engagement is seen as being synonymous with 'volunteering' and that such activities are being articulated as the 'model' for 'successful ageing' and negative judgements are made of those who do not take 'advantage' of the opportunity of 'old age' to participate in voluntary activity. This is, perhaps, not a trend yet evident in European gerontological discourse but it is noteworthy that older people constitute a large percentage of the voluntary sector 'workforce' as the following comments illustrate:

> I had a lot to do with men who had lost their jobs. They're all the same. They're very short on friends, real friends. Very short indeed. And when they come to the bowls club they come with marvellous ideas, I'm looking forward to this retirement, I've got the garden to do, I've got painting to do, I'll be fully occupied. But within three months they normally have a chat with me and say where do you think I can get a part-time job. [501: 4: 6]

> We've allowed ourselves to be overseers, it's sort of helping with the pastoral care in the community, visiting people, leading prayer and that sort of thing ... and that forces us to generate more social contact, not for our own benefit but to keep people in contact with the community and help with any problems that they might have. [203: 8: 1]

## 'Caring' activities

Included within the list of activities are two 'helping' roles – childcare and looking after someone who is frail or ill. Some 24 per cent reported that they had undertaken childcare activities in the previous month and 17 per cent that they had looked after someone else who was ill or frail (age not specified). Clearly these two sets of data illustrate the importance of older people in supporting children and the sick or frail within the community. Whilst it is not the focus of our investigation, it is clear that a key part of the 'social world' of older people is in caring and supporting others within their social network. Whilst we can only draw limited inferences from our study, our data broadly resonate with other research by illustrating the importance of older people in looking after children within their family network and the frail. As this extract illustrates, help flows across the generations are not simply from young to old:

> I spend a lot of time ... my granddaughter, she lives about 300 yards away and she's on her own with two children and she's had a rough time. ... so I spend a load of me time, she's got a house and things and I help out on occasion with clothes for the children and things because she's on next to nothing being a single parent. [406: 2: 4]

## Have levels of social participation changed over time?

How, if at all, has the pattern of social activities changed over time? We have already noted in Chapter 1 how the type of activities that older people have been asked if they engage in has changed across surveys in response to social changes and the development of a more affluent consumer-based society. Comparisons across studies are problematic because of variations across studies in the reference periods. As we argued earlier in this chapter, we should also not underestimate the importance of the place and the local cultural context in influencing the pattern of social engagement.

We can demonstrate the potential influence of time and space by reference to reported participation of older people in religious and faith-based activities in different community surveys. In our survey 29 per cent of participants reported attending church or some other faith-based activity, such as attending a mosque, in the previous month (see Table 3.4). This contrasts with the findings of Wenger (1984) who reported that 50 per cent of her sample attended church monthly, or perhaps more correctly in the location studied, chapel. However, this study is now over 20 years old and it is interesting to speculate if the same high levels of participation are still evident. Our data are comparable with the 26 per cent reported by Bond and Carstairs (1982) but double the 12 per cent reported by Townsend (1957).

It is, however, incontrovertible that church attendance and the social relationships that flow from this are very important in the social world of those who attend regularly, as the following illustrate.

> I am also very involved in the church now that I've got the time. Every Thursday I go to Mass in Stowmarket, and I am also involved in visiting, because the previous person who used to do it is very old. In fact they used to visit us when my husband was too ill for me to get to Mass but now I take communion to people who can't get to the church. He didn't want to go as much as I wanted to so I suppose now I am catching up on the things that I wanted to do. [301: 2: 29]

> Q: Do you think the church makes a difference then?

> A: Oh, a tremendous difference. Because immediately you move you are part of a large family. So you are part of a family and you meet people and however much you're on your own, out there are people who are there for you.

You're conscious that you belong to a big fellowship. As you say, you don't belong to the church for that reason, but the consciousness makes a big difference. You belong to something. The church is really the focal point of the community ... [404: 8: 2]

We get most of our social life through St Paul's Church, if there's anything going on there we go there. [206: 2: 16–17]

Interestingly, the church can also, via the pastoral and caring activities, provide a focus for those who do not attend services or who do not consider themselves to be believers:

And I do voluntary driving for the care, the church has a care society. I don't go to church I'm afraid, I should I know but I don't feel that I must go. But they have a care thing and I drive for them. I drive once or twice a week. I have two people to do tomorrow. That I take to the local hospitals or wherever it is they want to go to. I've got one to take to [name of town] tomorrow. So I enjoy doing that. [01: 06: 14–19]

## Later life and daily life

Thus far we have looked at distinct aspects of the social world of older people: contacts with family, neighbours and friends and engagement in the wider community. However, this is a very compartmentalised view of what, in reality, is a complex web of relationships and activities that take place within the specific context of older people's daily lives. In this final section we present qualitative data that focus on the activities in which older people participate on a daily basis and the impact these activities have on their lives. These accounts build a picture of day-to-day life and give a greater depth of understanding, not just to the individual activities undertaken in later life, but the reasons for the choice of these activities and how they are used to shape and structure lives which are not regulated by the requirement to participate in the formal labour market.

The tranche of literature addressing the 'quality of life' of older people (see Bowling, 1995 and 2005; Bond and Corner, 2004; Gabriel and Bowling, 2004a and 2004b) and the measurement of the quality of their lives focuses on the extent to which certain key factors are positively addressed in everyday life. Much has been written about the importance of: subjective satisfaction, physical environment, social environment, socio-economic factors, cultural factors, health status, personality and personal autonomy in relation to the daily lives of older people (Hughes, 1990; Bond and Corner, 2004). There is also a growing body of literature addressing the idea of 'successful' or 'positive' ageing (Baltes and Baltes, 1990; Bowling and Dieppe, 2005; Bowling and Iliffe, 2006). What is missing from these accounts, however, are the minutiae of daily life as it is lived and experienced by older people (Horgas et al., 1998). We know about the health of older people (both self-assessed and diagnosed), service use and social contact with friends, neighbours and relatives. We have paid far less attention, however, to what older people do on a day-to-day basis and how social participation and other activities are used to structure daily life; how much of 'daily life' is conducted in the private domain of home and how much in the 'outside' world. Indeed Bukov et al. (2002) argue that it is the unseen private world of home that dominates the daily life of older people. However, older people are not unique in the limited activity that has been expended upon studying daily life; it is only recently that sociologists have started to take an interest in this topic (Bennett and Watson, 2002; Silva and Bennet, 2003).

## Daily living

A large part of our participants's days were taken up with daily living: washing, dressing, housework, cooking, and shopping. These activities were often routinised to the extent that participants performed set tasks on set days, giving both a structure to the day and spreading out household tasks to make them more manageable. As we noted at the start of the chapter, there was a general discourse of 'slowing down' and reference to the fact that tasks such as cooking and cleaning take longer as people get older.

The idea of a fixed and fairly rigid routine echoes the findings of Percival (2002) in his study on the use and meanings given to domestic spaces, which highlights the importance of routine in daily activities. He suggests that, when eating alone, people cook similar meals at the same time each day and that the location of the meal and manner in which it is eaten (e.g. in front of the television or at the table) are rigidly adhered to on a daily basis. Participants, when asked to give a plan of activities for each day of the week, revealed set days for activities such as cleaning, baking and gardening. These activities could then be broken down according to which room they were taking place in and the times at which the activities were to take place. One of our participants, for example, always vacuumed the living room on a Tuesday and finished by 4:15pm so that she could be sitting with a cup of tea and a piece of cake by the time *Countdown* started at 4:30pm.

These extracts from the qualitative interviews illustrate how the pattern of days varies but carries vestiges of previous routines and habits such as getting up early.

> But if I'm home all day, ... well we get out of bed very early, because we've always been early risers so we get up at about half past five or six o'clock. Six probably. Erm, we have breakfast reasonably early, perhaps half past seven something like that. We read the paper perhaps, and then that there's always jobs around the house to be done, which we do. If I'm going to work that night I do have a sleep in the afternoon, I sort of sit on the settee and have a sleep. If I'm going out to work I usually leave at about half past seven although it depends because they start at different times. If not, erm ... we watch the television, read, just a normal sort of day merely nothing very exciting. [203: 1: 38–47]

> Well I'm up by seven o'clock. At five and 20 past seven this morning I was having my breakfast, my toast and cup of tea. Two slices of toast and marmalade. Then the cat came in and I had to feed the cat. Then I went straight and opened the bedroom window and turned the beds back so I could have some fresh air in. I do this is every morning, it is routine with me and then I go into the spare bedroom and pull the curtains back and then I go straight and washed the dishes. The dishes have to be washed and wiped and put away. Everything has to be put in its place. This is me, and I can't get out of it. I'm tidy, I'm too tidy. When I take a thing out it's got to be put back in its place. It's terrible isn't it?

> Q: So what do you do in the evenings then?

> A: I sit there in that chair. I've got my programmes. I like my quiz programmes. There's 15 to 1 and then I go straight from 15 to 1 to Ready Steady Cook, I like that, and then I go straight on to, Oh what's her name, they all laugh about her but she is such a nice person ... the missing link was her name, Anne Robinson. I love watching quizzes, this is what I'd do. I sit there in the evenings and I've got my soaps. And then about quarter to 10 I go and wash and clean my teeth and then I'm in bed by 10. I have a good night's sleep and then I'm ready to get up in the morning. And this is it. In the afternoon after I had my lunch I have a lie

down, and I'll lay down there for a solid hour or hour and a half and I'll go right off. And then I wake up and make myself a cup of tea and have a piece of sponge and then at about 5 o'clock I'll go and make my sandwiches. I always have ham sandwiches for tea. I shall look like a pig before long. And that's what I do. Mind I'm knitting all the time. [210: 33]

In addition to the development of the rhythm of each day there are activities and routines that mark out the different days of the week. For example, one participant reported:

Okay, we'll start with Monday. I feel that I've got to have a routine so that I know what I've got to do day in and day out. Monday is the day I go to Sainsburys to get my weekly shop. Tuesday is the day that I visit my wife. So that means that in the morning, obviously every day I have to cook my lunch, you know, that sort of thing, I go and see my wife on Tuesdays after lunch and I get there at about 2 o'clock ... so that's Tuesday. Wednesday ... is my bathroom washing day, I do the towels (laughs). I do two lots of washing. Thursday, like today, well that is housework and hoovering, dusting and so forth. Friday I go back to see my wife again. Saturday I do the bedroom wash if I can call it that, that's the sheets and pillow slips and that kind of thing. Also on Saturday I do part of the cooking. I do jam tarts on Saturday. If the weather is good in the afternoon or during the day I'll be out in the garden, I enjoy gardening. Erm ... Sunday is the morning when I cook the sponge, a victoria sponge. And then Monday I'm back again to the rounds you see. [205: 3: 7]

Other participants illustrate the importance of routines:

I see me sister every Saturday. One Saturday she comes to see me and the next Saturday I go and visit, you know. [407: 3: 7–8]

Another did their 'big' shop on Tuesday or Saturday:

Yes we tend to always shop on a Saturday morning, not for any particular reason, just that we always have done. [203: 4: 7–8]

Weekends were identified by differing routines – main meal at lunch on Sunday instead of the evening or attending church.

Sunday is fairly special to us because we attend Quaker meetings. We go out to a meeting on Sunday morning. Sometimes we go to another church perhaps, if we would like to meet with other Christian folk. [203: 2: 6–8]

Contact with family and friends also offers a way of structuring the pattern of the week, as the following illustrate:

... but my daughter, she comes by here Tuesdays and Thursdays, she also pops in sometimes at lunchtime. And Friday morning as she takes me into Bury shopping and then as I say she comes in on Sunday to pick up the baking that I've done for her and whatever, I do her mending because she's not very good with a needle! [306: 2:18–22]

I'll see my son and his family at least once a week and my daughter I'll see probably twice a week. We like to have lunch together at some point during the week, if we can manage it, just the two of us, rather than being surrounded by children and husbands and things. [502: 2: 20]

Always on a Sunday some part of the family comes. Saturdays I often go and visit my sister because she doesn't have very good health every week ... I'd see all five of my children at some point in time. [405: 3: 16]

... he [son] keeps Thursdays clear for me and he comes Sunday mornings and I'll spend the day there. And he'll have lunch with me Monday or Tuesday. And if he doesn't come over he'll ring come 7 or 8 o'clock. [603: 2: 46]

It is the time and space between the everyday tasks of daily life which cause problems for many of the older people interviewed. The cessation of full-time paid work or the children leaving home leaves a gap which needs to be filled. This is an area which has, with exception of studies examining adjustment to retirement and bereavement, been comparatively under-researched. The quest for many of our participants was to spend time in a pleasurable but also a productive way, a factor reflected in their comments. The focus was on developing interests and hobbies that would allow time to be filled productively and happily post-retirement. This was deemed important by people who were on their own, whether single, divorced or widowed, but equally by men who had stopped working full-time and had to find alternative ways to spend their time.

So many people used to say to me whatever you do don't retire. The secret is to keep interests. [504: 4: 49]

This was a view offered by participants who had jobs which they enjoyed, or which carried with them social relationships or status. The caveat was offered by one older man who commented:

> Well I hate to say this, but I am going to tell you the truth – when I was at work I never had much of a social life. [204: 6: 36]

This illustrates the problem: there is the need to develop interests and social networks before retirement, if possible, to make the transition less isolating. Not only is there a void in time, routine and structure to fill but, in the cases of predominantly male participants with long working hours, there are no existing social interests to fill it with. A lack of social activities and relationships outside of work prior to retirement was seen to predominantly affect men. One man reflected on the fact that, in his generation, men were more likely to work outside the home whilst women were more likely to work inside the home. Thus, as they aged, women were able to continue activities previously undertaken whilst men, on retirement, had to find alternative ways to occupy their time.

Maintaining interests was deemed important, but maintaining useful activities was stressed as even more essential. In some ways this echoes the points raised by Martinson and Minkler (2006) about civic engagement in later life being defined in terms of 'productive' activities such as volunteering.

> When you're working you're working for money. You've got family, you've got children. When that's all done you've then got to create other activities. [501: 7: 5]

> I think one of the awful things about getting older is that you feel that you're not wanted and can't do anything. [303: 4: 22]

The desire to feel useful, have a purpose for performing activities during the day and to be needed was a constant theme throughout the interviews. Retirement was seen as the catalyst for entering a new dimension of the life course. As such it was viewed with fear by some participants unsure how they would spend their time once this activity was no longer available.

> Actually I think that's something that worries me sometimes. The fact that I love working and I think I'm quite frightened of not working

really. And it does worry me – not being wanted, needed, you know. [203: 8: 43]

I've got no hobbies. I read, but I don't knit, I don't sew. Erm, I really haven't got any hobbies. I'm a bit apprehensive to retire, because what am I going to do? [701: 21–2]

This reflects the work of Phillipson (2002) where retirement is not feared solely as a loss of financial means but also as a loss of structure, friendship, community integration and usefulness. Thus, activities and routines have to be generated or expanded to fill those gaps.

The common theme running through the accounts was the need for productive ways of spending time – whether this be in the home, with friends and family or in the community, as this participant indicated:

It's surprising, if you are on your own and you've got time, I mean I don't mean to sound like a good Samaritan or something like that, but it's surprising what a lot of help you can give other people. Friends and family. For instance, a sister-in-law was moving, so what happens, I go round and stay with her help her to move. My son moved earlier on in the year and he asked whether I would come and help us move, you see. There's so much you can do when you've got the time, which I have now, to do other things for other people. And by doing that, you feel ... wanted, not exactly wanted but you feel a useful. [304: 12–19]

## Activities and hobbies

Abrams (1978), using figures from Social Trends 1985, suggested that:

the average retired person in Great Britain had on the average 24-hour day (including Saturday and Sunday) 10.3 hours of 'free time' (i.e., after 8.6 hours of sleep and 5.1 hours taken up with personal care and domestic work such as cooking, shopping, eating, washing); this was roughly four hours more 'free time' each day than that experienced by the average non-retired adult.

(Abrams, 1978: 30)

Abrams further suggested that over half of the 'free time' left to older people was spent watching television or listening to the radio, followed by time resting. Very little time was spent exercising, walking, playing sport or reading. More recent studies on the daily lives of older people include the Berlin Ageing Study (Horgas et al., 1998; Bukov et al., 2002) that asked people which activities they took part in and also the amount of time that they spent on each activity. In the three urban communities study carried out by Phillipson et al. (2001) participants were asked to rate the activities that they were most likely to do. The study found that reading was the most popular activity, followed by: gardening, watching television, walking, looking after the home, shopping and knitting. These results are very similar to our own. The following examples illustrate how these activities are integrated into people's daily lives but also show the breadth and diversity of activities that is sometimes obscured by the 'tick box' form of questioning about social activities used in social surveys.

> I used to be a dressmaker, part of my career with dressmaking and people tend to think that bit because you're retired you've got nothing to do and I get an abundance of things where one of the boys wants their trousers shortened or they want something mended. And I tend to spend the afternoon sewing or doing something of that nature. [305: 3: 13–16]

> Well I haven't started it yet but last winter I did an awful lot of walking. If I didn't go out anywhere else I'd go out and walk for two hours and I've got to start doing it again now, I mean through the summer I had the garden to do so I haven't been going out for long walks but when the weather gets like this I wrap up warm … [301: 6: 16–20]

> I've got a season ticket for the *** [football club], I go and watch the games. [204: 3: 24–5]

> I'm in the *** choir which practises once a week. We do a lot of concerts at the moment. We do a lot more at Christmas time with carols and things and we go to *** for rehearsal which is a fair few miles each way so it's quite a way for choir practice. [101: 2: 43–6]

Gardening was one of the most common activities reported by participants (see Table 3.4), which ties in with the work of Phillipson et al. (2001b) where gardening was rated second only to reading as the most popular activity. Gardening was seen to have a number of benefits. It provided exercise, a creative outlet, a link to a growing, changing landscape and a means of providing a routine or timetable for the day or season.

> I never get bored. I can always, well I'll do the gardening or do some decorating – working in the garden, yes I can push myself in the garden

and it doesn't do any harm as long as I'm careful. I mean until I retired I never did anything. [506: 4: 20]

Here gardening represents a sea change in activity rather than simply in the amount of time spent doing an activity.

I suppose you could say that on an average weekday I nearly always spend part of the time outside, somehow I don't like to be housebound. An average weekday would probably be something just messing about in the garden. It might be cutting the lawn, or keeping the hedges in trim, that sort of thing. [705: 4: 47]

Gardening was also seen as a social activity.

If we're at home we do like to go somewhere. We go out and think we ought to do that, you know, maybe we go to the garden centre. This year we joined the horticultural society and so we've been to all sorts of places. [702: 4: 47]

Two men were members of horticultural societies, two women were part of groups which visited famous gardens, and a number of others talked about occasional group trips to gardens in their local area as part of social groups, women's groups or church groups. Involvement in gardening, like other interests, can lead into a much greater form of community involvement.

I'm a vice president of the *** horticultural society and I've always been interested in gardening so I do a fair bit of voluntary work still for them. I've been the chairman, I've been the treasurer, I've been the president. And I still distribute the newsletter. We do a monthly newsletter which we distribute to members. I still distribute a lot of those because I still drive the car. And that takes, you know, about a day a week. [204: 2: 15–19]

The temporal nature of gardening, however, goes some way to explaining the temporal nature of the daily lives of older people, which change significantly with the seasons.

Normally I like to get out in the garden but it's been far too wet for weeks now. So I've been sewing things – and making things! Doing my daughter's mending. [306: 2: 1]

I mean I still like to garden, but I must admit with this horrible weather we've had, it's been so terrible and it's very heavy clay round here so at the moment the garden is absolutely on top. I stripped out the bedding plants in the front there and I haven't even put anything back in yet. And I've got tons of bulbs to plant but I've been waiting for the weather to make the soil workable again, you know. So I'm miles behind with that. But that's how I spend my time. [204: 2: 44]

As this final quote shows, gardening is not just an activity but a means of structuring time.

## Pets

Pets also generate activity as they need to be fed, exercised and generally cared for.

We've got a reason to go out now you see. We take him out in the morning for an hour and then last thing at night we take him out for another walk for a good hour before we settle for the night. So you're all getting more exercise. [407: 4: 19]

When I'm walking the dogs I will always see somebody, and we have, every two months we have a get together, all the dog walking friends. We go and have lunch. [703: 4: 16]

Pet ownership fulfils many needs. It can provide a means of getting exercise, a structure for the day, a feeling of being needed and useful, a means of generating social contact and social contact in itself. The friendships forged through meeting on a daily basis whilst walking dogs both allowed for social contact and the possibility of making new friends, and also gave a structure to the day. Pet ownership has also been examined as a possible protective factor in reducing loneliness in older people and as a companion (Ory and Goldberg, 1983) and as an opportunity for conversation. However, the research evidence supporting 'animal-assisted therapy' is limited and inconclusive (Filan and Llewellyn-Jones, 2006; Banks and Banks, 2002). However, within a community setting older people walking their dogs have a route into conversation with others and an opportunity for exercise!

Pet ownership can also lead to a more external involvement in voluntary activities. For example:

I'm very much involved, as I say, with this animal charity. And at least one day a week I go over and spend my time helping to sort things out for the charity. You know, sorting out bric-a-brac and washing jumble and that sort of thing. [304: 2: 13–15]

## Community-based activities

Relationships with friends could also be extended into the community and linked to community-based activities. The nature of the types of activities in which older people are engaging within the community is diverse and changing. This is a theme which has been addressed by a variety of writers looking at the changing nature of ageing and of later life. In his book *Ageing and Popular Culture* Andrew Blaikie (1999) assesses the ways in which the ageing process has been portrayed across time and suggests that processes of ageing, such as full-time education, are no longer solely chronologically determined. Older people are now engaging in activities previously thought the domain of the young. He suggests:

> We have moved, then, beyond the era of progressive, linear stages of development, where age is assumed – 'naturally' – to determine a child's behaviour and how it relates to adults. What this demonstrates is that age-appropriate behaviour is a system of roles that have been socially constructed.
>
> (Blaikie, 1999 : 170)

If this is the case, then it should be demonstrable through an examination of the actions and activities of older people. The increased numbers of older people entering education, the development of the University of the Third Age, the growth of grey power (as demonstrated by the recent cases of pensioner protests in relation to council tax) and the emergence of older people – Third Agers – as a key focus of consumer society, all point to the social construction of 'age-appropriate' roles. Roles once considered solely as the domain of the young are now not only open to, but actively recruiting, older people.

The wider community provides a range of activities through which day-to-day life may be filled. Our participants gave a range of examples of community-based activities in which they were involved, including: clubs, voluntary work, church work and the University of the Third Age. Social clubs were mentioned by a number of participants. They were most commonly associated with a particular interest such as music, horticulture or the church. Three women also talked about membership of the University of the Third Age, a forum for learning and developing interests but also a social event and way of making and meeting friends. Davey (2002) has examined the growth of education and re-skilling in mid or later life as part of what she terms an 'active ageing' approach. This links with the idea that older people are engaging in activities which stretch their minds as well as enabling them to participate in society. Huber and Skidmore (2003) suggest that the phenomenon of post-retirement education is one that is expanding and that it will grow significantly when the 'baby-boomer' generation retires as many of them are expressing an interest in education, and, more specifically, education which is not tied to the workplace.

Church membership could act to make Sundays the social focus of the week rather than the low point as far as social interaction was concerned. Church was also seen as a means of generating a social life:

> Our greatest involvement, I think, is with the church. Every one is so ordinary and nice. And if you go in and have not been for a while it's like going back into the family. And they have good things at Christmas, and they have barn dances. It's a very alive church, so you see, our social life is really in the church. [206: 3: 22]

The importance of voluntary work as a way of spending time and remaining useful was also stressed in a wider context as we noted earlier. In these contexts volunteering can be understood both as a way of generating activity and spending time but also as a way of extending reciprocity, being useful and giving something back. Voluntary activity is recognised as providing both a 'social purpose' and as a form of 'pressure group', giving older people a collective forum for change. The next two decades, however, may see a drop in the numbers of older people engaging in voluntary work as the 'baby boomers' reach old age. Huber and Skidmore (2003) chart a significant rise in the number of older people undertaking self-employment after they have retired from traditional employment, and suggest that these numbers will continue to grow as the nature of employment is changed by the baby-boom generation.

> With 50.5 per cent of baby boomers claiming they would 'rather be a self-employed entrepreneur than a 9–5 employee' (Mori Social Values 1999) we might see an unprecedented rise in older people wanting to use

the time and resources afforded by their retirement to start their own company.

(Huber and Skidmore, 2003: 58)

In this chapter we have explored the patterns of social relations through our survey data of contact with family, friends and neighbours, wider social participation in the community and everyday activities. We have used extracts from the qualitative interviews with some of our participants to illustrate the experience of social relations in later life. Our data suggest that for many in their Third Age there is increasing involvement and participation in social life but as people age, chiefly those in their 80s and 90s, patterns of social relations change with the loss of close friends and relatives, particularly life-long partners and confidants, and with functional impairment. It would appear that it is the final years of life that increase the risk of loneliness and isolation because of the changing nature of social relations. In the next chapter we explore our participants' experience of loneliness and isolation and the meaning this has for their lives.

# 4

# Experiences of loneliness

In the previous chapter we examined the broad context of older people's social relations: relationships with their family, friends, neighbours and the wider social world. We also explored how social relations and activities were central to the rhythm of daily life. In this chapter we focus more specifically upon the experiences and perceptions of loneliness – a topic that has been studied in terms of both empirical research (Heinrich and Gullone, 2006) and literature (Nilsson et al., 2006). For many people loneliness is seen as an integral, inevitable and virtually universal aspect of later life. Indeed this is one of the most enduring and potentially pernicious of all stereotypes of old age and later life.

A recent survey in the United States (National Council on the Aging, 2002) revealed that 38 per cent of people aged under 65 years and 84 per cent of people aged 65 years or over thought that loneliness was 'a very or somewhat serious' problem for older people. However, only 21 per cent of survey respondents aged 65 years or over thought that it was 'a very or somewhat serious' problem for them. This contrasts to an ICM telephone poll in Britain commissioned by the BBC, which found that only nine per cent of respondents of all ages thought loneliness was a problem of old age. The ICM poll respondents focused much more upon health (35 per cent) and income and finances (26 per cent) as the major problems of later life (BBC, 2004). However, a MORI poll commissioned by the Help the Aged British Gas partnership in 2000 concluded 'that nearly one million older people are acutely isolated and over one million people aged 65 and over (12%) feel trapped in their own home' (Ipsos MORI, 2000). In a separate poll for *Independent Age* MORI found that fears about loneliness in old age decreased with age from 46 per cent of younger people (aged 15–24 years) to 25 per cent among older people (aged 65 years or over) (Ipsos MORI, 2005). The way that questions are asked in these polls will often reinforce society's stereotypes. The way headline results are presented and the media response to poll conclusions may equally reinforce society's stereotypes.

In Britain loneliness and isolation have become an important issue for advocacy organisations such as Help the Aged which 'is an international charity fighting to free disadvantaged older people from poverty, isolation and neglect' (Help the Aged, 2007). They have organised awareness raising and fundraising campaigns like HUG (Help Unite Generations) and One is the Saddest Number. The importance of advocacy organisations in raising the awareness of key issues of later life to disadvantaged older people cannot be overvalued. However, an inevitable consequence of the campaigns run by advocacy organisations in the UK and North America is that they reinforce this negative stereotype of later life – that isolation and loneliness are an inevitable part of old age – and by so doing may undermine another goal of these organisations, which is to eradicate ageism.

How accurate are these stereotypes about loneliness and isolation in later life? In this chapter we report in depth how loneliness is experienced in later life using both survey data and the qualitative interviews to highlight the key issues. In Chapter 5 we report the experiences and perceptions of social isolation and exclusion.

## Loneliness in later life

As we discussed in Chapter 2, for a construct like loneliness, which is contested in terms of its theoretical foundation and operationalisation, there are numerous scales and approaches available towards the measurement of this social phenomena as well as the use of indirect measures such as marital status (Friedlander et al., 1995). Conceptually we identified two different approaches to measuring loneliness. The one-dimensional approach views loneliness as a single phenomenon that varies by experienced intensity. In contrast, the multidimensional approach conceptualises loneliness as a multifaceted phenomenon and one that often provides both an overall score and identifies distinct components of loneliness encapsulated within specific indices. Most of the measurement scales are 'indirect' in that they do not explicitly mention the topic of interest. This is unlike the single-question approach that seeks a participant's assessment of loneliness using a Likert-type scale with varying degrees of sophistication in the level of response. Here the focus is upon identifying the intensity of the experience rather than identifying the underlying constructs. A key objection to the use of the single-question 'self-rating' scale is that it requires participants to 'admit' their loneliness and so participants may downplay their responses for fear of compromising their sense of self-worth.

In this study we used the single-question approach, as one objective of our project was to compare our survey results with those from previous British studies. We were intrigued to try to establish if loneliness is more (or less) prevalent in contemporary generations of older people than earlier generations. Our question is shown in Table 4.1 and is compared with those used by both Sheldon (1948) and Townsend (1957) and with other studies that have used this approach. The common characteristic of the questions used in the surveys reported is that they require participants to rate directly their current

**Table 4.1** Self-rating loneliness scales used in various studies

| Author | Measure |
| --- | --- |
| Sheldon (1948) | Are you very lonely, lonely at times or never lonely? |
| Townsend (1957) | Are you very, sometimes or never lonely? |
| Shanas et al. (1968) | Are you lonely often, sometimes, rarely, never? |
| Bond and Carstairs (1982) | Are you lonely never, sometimes, often? |
| Jones et al. (1985) | Are you lonely never, sometimes, often, always? |
| Samuelsson et al. (1998) | Are you lonely never, sometimes, often, always? |
| Holmen and Furukawa (2002) | Do you experience loneliness, always, often, sometimes, seldom, never? |
| Harris et al. (2003) | Are you lonely never, sometimes, often, always? |
| Jylhä (2004) | Are you lonely often, sometimes, never? |
| (Victor et al., 2005b) | Do you always feel lonely, often feel lonely, sometimes feel lonely, never feel lonely? |

levels of loneliness. There is a clear and unambiguous mention of the topic that we are interested in. However, there is a variation in the wording of questions including subtle differences in the tense, for example: 'Do you ....', 'Are you ....' or 'Would you say ....'. There is also variation in the degree of gradation of response categories. It is not clear as to the genesis of this question. The earliest reference found thus far is in Sheldon (1948) but it is not clear from the text whether that study created the question or whether it derived from elsewhere. Certainly there is no information provided upon the development and testing of the question. Whilst it has face validity in that it is understood by survey participants, with few studies reporting missing data for this question, there is no evidence to date that it was ever subject to any developmental testing before being used by Sheldon (1948) and subsequently others.

The use of a single question is pragmatic but there has been some work undertaken on the validity and reliability of single-question self-rating measures to test their value as a measurement tool. Such a 'simple' question has considerable appeal both for the survey researchers, trying to reduce the length of their questionnaires, and service providers seeking out a screening tool that can be used effectively within a service delivery context. Therefore for pragmatic reasons it is important to develop brief, valid and reliable measures such as the reduced UCLA scale or the short form of the New York University loneliness scale. The latter uses three questions to assess how often participants felt lonely, how lonely they felt and how lonely they were in comparison to those of their own age (Kielcot-Glaser et al., 2003). Longer scales, such as those containing 60 items, have fallen out of favour with researchers (Solano, 1980).

Loucks undertook an evaluation of the Bradley loneliness scale in the United States and demonstrated that the loneliness scale showed construct validity by its ability to discriminate between those who were depressed or anxious. It also demonstrated poor 'self-concept' and other related emotional states (Loucks, 1980). Similarly, Russell et al. (1978) and Cramer and Barry (1999) indicated that self-reported current loneliness states were correlated with scores on the UCLA scale and the Social and Emotional Loneliness Scale for Adults (SELSA). However, both of these evaluation studies were undertaken with university students rather than older people. In these studies the self-rating scales were used to demonstrate the face validity of the indices being tested rather than being used as a means of supporting the use of self-rating scales. However, they do lend some support for the use of the self-rating scales.

## The extent of loneliness in later life

As we have reported elsewhere the majority of participants in our survey, 61 per cent, rated themselves as never lonely, 31 per cent as 'sometimes' lonely, five per cent as often lonely and two per cent as always lonely (Victor et al., 2005b). This finding, that the majority of older people do not experience loneliness, is consistent with the majority of studies undertaken in Britain (Table 4.2) and also does not seem to be dependent upon the mode of data collection (postal surveys as compared with direct interviews). For example, the survey by Harris and colleagues (Harris et al., 2003), using a postal survey, reported a very similar prevalence of loneliness as the direct interview surveys such as ours and those undertaken by Shanas and colleagues (1968) or Townsend (1957). Indeed Lauder et al. (2006a) suggest that loneliness is relatively stable within the older population. In terms of the levels of 'severe' loneliness, the 'outliers' from the general pattern, with reported loneliness rates of 16 per cent, are those conducted in three deprived areas (Scharf et al., 2002) and inner London (Bowling and Browne, 1991; Prince et al., 1997).

## How does loneliness change over time?

A key purpose of our study was to establish how the experience of loneliness has (or has not) changed for different cohorts of older people in Britain. The rationale for this was to examine the popular assumption that changes in the domestic and family structures of older people have resulted in an increased prevalence of loneliness amongst contemporary cohorts of older people. In this analysis we make comparisons using data from different cross-sectional studies building on an earlier analysis by Victor and colleagues (Victor et al., 2002). However, this is not a longitudinal analysis of individual change.

In Table 4.2 we can see that the relationship between the percentage describing themselves as 'sometimes' or 'never' lonely has been changing over time, especially in studies using rating scales where respondents choose from a selection of closed questions with relative

**Table 4.2** Prevalence of loneliness – selected UK studies (%)

| Date | Author | Study area | Sample size | Never lonely | Sometimes | Very/often lonely/always lonely |
|------|--------|-----------|-------------|--------------|-----------|----------------------------------|
| 1948 | (Sheldon, 1948)≠ | Wolverhampton | 400+ | 79 | 13 | 8 |
| 1957 | (Townsend, 1957)≠ | London | 203 | 72 | 22 | 5 |
| 1966 | (Tunstall, 1966) | 4 centres | 526 | 66 | 25 | 9 |
| 1968 | (Shanas et al., 1968)≠ | Great Britain | 2483 | 72 | 21 | 7 |
| 1978 | (Hunt, 1978) | England | 2622 | | | 13-response to 'open' question |
| 1982 | (Bond and Carstairs, 1982)≠ | Clackmannan | 1000+ | 74 | 19 | 7 |
| 1984 | (Wenger, 1984)≠ | North Wales | 683 | 76 | 19 | 5 |
| 1985 | (Jones et al., 1985)≠ | South Wales | 654 | 76 | 19 | 5* |
| | | Mid Wales | 628 | 84 | 14 | 2* |
| 1989 | (Qureshi and Walker, 1989) | Sheffield | 306 | | | 12** |
| 1991 | (Bowling et al., 1991) | Hackney | 1053 | | | 16 |
| | | Essex | 288 | | | 8 |
| 1997 | (Prince et al., 1997) | Gospel Oak (district of London) | 654 | 61 | 13 | 16 |
| 2002 | (Scharf et al., 2002) | 3 deprived inner city areas of England | 595 | 40 | 44 | 16 |
| 2003 | (Harris et al., 2003) | South London | 1214 | 52 | 39 | 9 |
| 2005 | (Victor et al., 2005b)≠ | Great Britain | 999 | 61 | 31 | 7 |

Note: ≠These studies use similar single-question self-rating scales (see Table 4.1)

133

frequency options. A literature review of loneliness scales by Pepper (1981) revealed that the respondents' interpretations of the term 'sometimes' are variable; with many people understanding it to be about 20 per cent of the time, while others understood it to mean about half the time. Furthermore, in this review there was also overlap between the terms 'rarely' and 'sometimes', adding further response error. Whilst this review was undertaken some time ago it seems unlikely that the central point of the argument, the lack of precision of the intermediate loneliness rating categories, will have changed. Schaeffer (1991) recommends that relative frequency responses currently used in many scales are replaced by absolute frequency response options, such as 'everyday' or 'once a week'. The use of absolute frequency response options increases the possibility that comparisons between groups would be valid reflections of the concept, and not caused by differences in how groups interpret the response option terms. Variations in how the term 'sometimes' is interpreted may explain some of the observable increase in this response category over time (see Table 4.2). However, the percentage defined as 'seriously' lonely seems remarkably constant both historically and across the countries of Northern Europe, North America and Australia.

Table 4.2 also provides an illustration of the variations in the extent of loneliness identified when using multidimensional scales and indices rather than single-question self-rating scales. The study of loneliness in North Wales by Wenger et al. (1996) provides the opportunity to compare the results from a single-question self-rating scale with an eight-item uni-dimensional scale. As Table 4.2 reveals the single-question self-rating scale does not alter the broad pattern of the distribution of responses but does increase the percentage of people classed in the intermediate and severe categories and decreases the 'non' lonely group.

## Variations in loneliness across countries

How do levels of loneliness compare with those reported in other countries? This is a difficult question to answer as the meaning of terms such as 'loneliness' is highly culturally (and possibly temporally) specific. Nevertheless determining if loneliness is a universal element of old age and later life is a question of interest to gerontologists (de Jong-Gierveld and Havens, 2004). Surveys of loneliness have been undertaken in Australia (Flood, 2005), Europe (van Tilburg et al., 1998), China (Dong et al., 2007; Liu and Guo, 2007), Taiwan (Wang et al., 2001), Nepal (Chalise et al., 2007), with migrant groups (Kim, 1999), and with those resident in institutions (Drageset, 2004). Making comparisons of the extent of loneliness across different countries is rendered more problematic because of the variation in measures used. Using studies that have (mostly) used self-rating questions and/or are conducted in Western countries, Table 4.3 demonstrates that there seems to be some consistency in levels of reported loneliness in samples of older people drawn from northern European, North American and Australasian samples. Again there seems to be consistent finding of about 15–30 per cent of survey participants reporting any experience of loneliness. Consistently most older people do not experience this problem.

However, in addition as Jylhä (2004) has noted, loneliness is very culturally and temporally specific and, perhaps, this is not well illustrated by the above table. One way to examine this more rigorously is to undertake explicitly comparative studies across different countries using identical methods. There are a few studies that have applied common methods of measurement in differing locations. Victor et al. (2005a) reports that using a self-report measure eight per cent of those aged 65 years and over in Perth (Western Australia) were often or always lonely, 33 per cent sometimes lonely and 62 per cent never lonely – rates virtually identical to those in the UK.

Within Europe Jylhä and Jokela (1990), Imamoglu et al. (1993), van Tilburg et al. (1998) and van Tilburg et al. (2004) have reported a 'north-south' divide in loneliness across Europe. Levels of loneliness are lowest in northern Europe and increase as we move to the southern Mediterranean countries. For example, the European Study of Adult Well-being – a six-country study of adults aged 50 years or over – documented self-reported rates of loneliness of between four per cent and twelve per cent in Sweden, Austria, Luxemburg, Holland, the UK and Italy (see Burholt et al., 2003 for full details). Walker and Maltby (1997) reported rates of loneliness up to nine per cent in Denmark, Germany, Holland and the UK; 10–15 per cent for Belgium, France, Luxembourg, Ireland, Spain and Italy, and 36 per cent in Greece. Explicit comparisons of loneliness across markedly differing cultures are even rarer. Victor and Yang (2006) have compared levels of

**Table 4.3** Levels of loneliness – selected non-UK studies

| Author | Location | Sample size/ age group | Loneliness |
|---|---|---|---|
| Shanas et al. (1968) | USA | 2417 | 9% often lonely |
| Shanas et al. (1968) | Denmark | 2436 | 4% often lonely |
| Hall and Havens (1999) | Manitoba Canada | 1868 65+ | 16% not lonely, 38% somewhat lonely and 45% quite lonely |
| Holmen and Furukawa (2002) | Sweden | 1702 | 36% any degree of loneliness |
| Steed et al. (2007) | Perth, Western Australia | 353 65+ | 7% always/often lonely, 32% sometimes lonely |
| Jylhä (2004) | Tampere, Finland | 787 aged 65+ | 8% often lonely, 27% sometimes lonely |
| Tiikkainen et al. (2004) | Finland | 207 aged 80+ | 5% often lonely |
| Stek et al. (2004) | Leiden, Holland | 500 aged 85+ | 19% any degree of loneliness |
| Tiikkainen and Heikkinen (2005) | Finland | 133 aged 85 | 8% lonely (often/ always) |
| Treacy et al. (2005) | Eire | 683 aged 65+ | 12% 'socially lonely', 7% experience family loneliness |
| Routasalo et al. (2006) | Finland | 4113 aged 75+ | 39% any degree of loneliness |

loneliness between Britain and China and reported that loneliness in China, as measured by a variant of the 'self-report' measure, increased 15.6 per cent to 29.6 per cent between 1992 and 2000. This level of reported loneliness broadly fits the pattern demonstrated in Table 4.3.

However, we must remember that our data, and the majority of other work across varying settings and societies, indicates that the majority of older people do not feel lonely. It is important that we retain this perspective when we are examining in more detail the other aspects of loneliness such as definitions, causes and consequences. The majority views of older people are summarised in the following quote:

Do I ever feel lonely? I don't honestly think I do. [303: 4: 1–6]

## Public and private accounts of loneliness

As was noted earlier, a key objection, at least in theory, to the use of self-rating scales is that they require participants to 'admit' that they are experiencing a potentially stigmatising and compromising social phenomena. It is, therefore, sometimes argued that participants do not give a true account of their feelings of loneliness by either not reporting the experience or downgrading the intensity of the experience. Indeed a recurrent theme within the 'loneliness measurement' literature is the debate about asking direct and indirect types of questions and the degree to which they will reveal only the 'public account' rather than the participants' true feelings. Indeed, loneliness is not something one might 'admit to one's friends' let alone a stranger arriving to interview you, as this comment suggests:

I think it's a very difficult thing to quantify ... because we're talking about a friend of ours, who, it's sad for her because she does obviously feel very lonely although she wouldn't admit it I think. [203: 5: 42]

We can go some way to examining this issue by comparing the self-rating of loneliness given by those who participated in our qualitative study. We can compare their interviews with their initial rating. This revealed that for the 45 participants in the qualitative interviews there was considerable consistency across the two forms of interview. Twenty participants rated themselves as 'not lonely' in the survey interview and did not demonstrate a discourse of loneliness in the qualitative interview; similarly, 19 rated themselves as lonely, in varying degrees, in the survey interview and talked openly about their loneliness in the qualitative interview. However, there was some discordance with five people reporting and talking about their loneliness in the qualitative interview but not in the survey interview and one for whom the opposite was the case. This is obviously not a rigorous evaluation of the self-rating question but suggests that it has some face validity.

However, further work is required to consider the discontinuities of response which may have reflected changed circumstances because there was a six to nine-month gap between the two interviews. Given the length of time between the two data-collection points the similarity of response would seem impressive.

Another perspective upon this issue is to compare levels of loneliness generated using different types of measures (direct questions compared with unidimensional and multidimensional scales) and different methods of data collection (direct interviews compared with postal surveys). Recently Victor and colleagues (Victor et al., 2005b) have compared the use of a self-report measure of loneliness with the UCLA and de Jong scales in a postal survey of older people living in Perth, Australia and drawn comparisons with data collected through face-to-face interview. This was not a true evaluation of the psychometric properties of the different measures but rather an evaluation of their practical use in a postal survey, a comparison of their acceptability to older people and a test of their effectiveness as classificatory or screening devices. It also enabled us to start to address the importance of 'mode effects' upon data collected concerning sensitive and potentially compromising or threatening aspects of old age and later life.

The exercise revealed that there were specific problems of item non-response with the UCLA and de Jong scales, which were accentuated in the postal survey compared with the face-to-face interviews. In the postal survey 353 older people returned questionnaires. Item omission prevented the calculation of the de Jong scale for 53 respondents and of the UCLA scale for 17 respondents (15 per cent and 5 per cent of respondents respectively). In comparison only ten respondents (3 per cent) did not respond to the single-question self-rating scale.

This illustrates why short-form versions of measurement scales, which have the potential for limiting respondent fatigue and item non-response, are attractive to researchers as the successive shortening of the UCLA scale illustrates. Levels of 'non-response' to the single-question self-rating scale are generally low. However, the study by Hall and Havens (1999) in Manitoba Canada had an unusually high level of non-response to their single-question self-rating scale with 465 out of 1868 participants (25 per cent) not responding to the question that asked them to rate themselves as not, somewhat or quite lonely. Perhaps the distinction between somewhat and quite lonely was problematic.

Comparing the estimates of loneliness generated from the survey interview with those derived from postal surveys in Perth, Australia (Victor et al., 2005b) and south London (Victor et al., 2002) reveals considerable similarities across the three studies. First, non-response to the single-question self-rating scale was marginal in our direct interval survey (three respondents did not answer the question) and minimal in the two postal surveys (4/245 in south London and 4/353 in the Perth survey). Second, the prevalence of risk factors for loneliness such as widowhood (28% in the ESRC study, 40% in south London and 395 in Perth), gender (48%, 48% and 53% respectively) and living alone (31%, 29% and 37% respectively) were broadly similar across these three studies. This comparison therefore suggests that these estimates of the prevalence of loneliness are robust and not dependent on the mode of survey data-collection method: postal self-completed or structured face-to-face interview.

From the Perth study direct comparison of the three measures gave very similar estimates of the extent of loneliness with eight per cent rating themselves as very or often lonely and nine per cent classed as severely or very severely lonely on the de Jong scale. However, the measures performed rather differentially in their evaluation of the intermediate and 'never or not lonely' groups. Using the self-report measure 32 per cent rated themselves as sometimes lonely and 62 per cent as never lonely compared with 39 per cent classified as moderately lonely on the de Jong scale and 52 per cent as not lonely.

So we may conclude that the self-report and scale measures concur in their identification of those at the two extremes of the loneliness distribution – those who are definitely lonely and those who are not. However, there was variability across the measures in the classification of those in the 'intermediate' categories, which probably reflects where category boundaries are drawn.

## Temporal aspects of loneliness

A key theme of this chapter is the dynamic nature of loneliness. Both the survey and qualitative data highlight the importance of the temporal dimension of loneliness. In the survey, of those who reported sometimes, often or always feeling lonely, 54 per cent also reported experiencing loneliness at specific times. This could relate to specific times of the year, seasons or days of the week, evenings, weekends and holiday periods being the most problematic. Sundays were particularly difficult for people who were not active members of churches.

I suppose you feel lonely at the strangest times really. It isn't when you're sort of sat on your own and things like that, it's something that crops up on television and all of a sudden there's nobody there to pass a comment to. [602: 5: 23]

... yes. Saturday is my rest day, I think because most people are tied up with their families. Strangely enough Sunday doesn't bother me. Saturday seems to be the worst day. Which is peculiar. [602: 2: 34]

... Sunday I don a tracksuit and do the cleaning of the house and dig out all the corners. Sunday to me is the day when I don't usually go visiting because everybody has got their husbands and partners and families around them. [305: 5: 11]

Occasionally, as I say, particularly over bank holiday times and things like that, when everybody you look at seems to be in couples or families. [305: 6: 28]

You can be very lonely, yes, particularly in the winter. I don't go out as much in the winter obviously and if the roads are treacherous and the paths are treacherous I probably shouldn't go out at all because I'd be scared of falling. Touch wood, I've never fallen out of doors yet but a lot of my friends have. [202: 6: 41]

Oh yes, I feel lonely sometimes in the winter. Particularly in the winter, you feel lonely because there's rain outside and there's a limit to your reading and you're reluctant to go out. [501: 6: 9]

## Changes in loneliness for individuals

In the survey ten per cent of participants reported that they were less lonely than they were 10 years before, 23 per cent were more lonely and 77 per cent reported no change in their perception of loneliness. This suggests that, over a decade, 30 per cent perceived a change in their experience of loneliness, but for the majority there was no change. This analysis reveals a group of older people for whom levels of loneliness may be decreasing. This runs entirely counter to the general stereotype of loneliness in later life that changes in loneliness can only be for the worse. The participants' responses to this question therefore highlight the potential fluctuations in individuals' perception of their past experience of loneliness and that levels of loneliness at an individual level can both improve or deteriorate. Using a combination of responses to the questions examining current levels of loneliness and changes over the past decade, five distinct trajectories of loneliness across the life course were identified:

◆ Those for whom loneliness is perceived as an unchanged and constant feature of life.

◆ Those for whom loneliness in later life is a new experience.

◆ Those for whom the experience of loneliness is perceived as increasing.

◆ Those for whom loneliness is perceived as decreasing.

◆ Those who never experience loneliness.

In the qualitative interviews we were able to explore retrospectively these trajectories in depth. From the analysis of the transcripts of the qualitative interviews three theoretically grounded categories of the experience of loneliness in later life emerged. These are regenerative, degenerative and the existential. We describe these categories further and illustrate them with the comments of our participants and then consider how well these pathways categorise our survey group. This illustrates the value of a mixed-methods approach whereby insights and typologies developed from qualitative data can be applied to the survey population and be used to inform and develop the statistical analysis of the survey data.

## Decreasing levels of loneliness

The regenerative trajectory identifies those for whom there is a reduction in loneliness across the life course. There were two distinct aspects of this trajectory. First for a subgroup of single, never-married women, it was the peer pressure when younger that made them feel lonely. As one of our participants explained, she was put under pressure to establish relationships and was made to feel inadequate because she had chosen not to marry. With age there was less pressure and she was able to develop coping strategies for her life alone. This meant that she became less lonely as she grew older, and more able to cope with being alone, and with other people's opinions of the fact that she was alone.

Q: Do you every feel lonely?

A: Yes I think I do sometimes ... It's something you learn to accept ...

Q: And is it something that you've only noticed recently or something that you've always been aware of?

A: Oh no, I would say it was worse when I was younger.

Q: So what do you think causes this loneliness then?

A: .. I don't know really ... I think it gets less as you get older, as one gets less sensitive [laughs] and also one learns to cope with so many different situations, you know, that it gets easier. [106: 5: 6]

For another group of participants their experiences of loneliness were caused by a specific traumatic event of some kind – usually the loss of a partner, or the onset of severe, restrictive health problems. Over the course of time, the individual adapted to the loss of a partner, limited health or impaired mobility and modified their daily lives to the new circumstances in which they found themselves. They gradually became less lonely. This pathway was particularly common amongst men and women who had been widowed or divorced for a number of years and had been able to adapt their lives and develop new friendships and relationships in response to their loss.

I was widowed almost two years ago and of course that was very difficult because I'd nursed my husband at home, and of course he was blind for years before that so everything did close in on us a lot. But since then ... erm ... OK, so I've joined the *** Town Women's Guild, I only went on one meeting and I went on one trip to ***. So I did go to evening classes and took an intermediate thing on word processing because I wanted to update my system. Apart from that I've done various classes and I've been helping my daughter who's a recovering alcoholic, but we don't talk about that ... I've got the dog who I walk twice a day, in this weather that's great ... I do a lot in the garden ... Basically I suppose I'm a lot better off that I was last time you interviewed me, I'm very lucky. [507: 1: 3]

Q: So how long have you known your dance partner?

A: 15 years, and she just happened to come down to St Peter's Church and came to a dance and my wife made friends with her, used to go on holidays together, and she taught her dancing. And so that's how we met. And then when my wife died, of course, she was very good because she used to be in hospitals as an orderly, and so she was used to looking after people. And then when she was ill, the last two years she was a great boon to me, looking after her and helping me. So when that happened she said we might as well carry on, she said, because we've been friends all this time. So that's how I met her, we've stayed together ever since. They were the best of friends her and my wife. And she's been a great help to me. Because it gets me out, that's the point, so I don't watch television all the time. [105: 4: 34]

It took me a long time to get used to it when I was on my own at first. When I first came in this flat, for two years I wasn't happy. I thought I would never get used to it. But after two years I remember thinking one day oh I must get home, and that's the first point where I thought of it as home. Bearing in mind that I had had a nervous breakdown. You see after my husband died everyone said how marvellous I was, I kept up because I had three girls at home. It was after they left home. Then I was really on my own and it really hit me. Twenty-three years ago this November John died. Very sudden it was, very, very sudden. I was 46. [405: 4: 12]

## Increasing levels of loneliness: the degenerative pathway

In contrast the degenerative trajectory describes a pattern of increasing levels of loneliness across the life course. This is where, for a significant number of people, their mobility, social circumstances, health, financial situations, etc., conspire to result in a situation where they become increasingly lonely as they get older. Fifteen of those we interviewed in depth suggested that they were more lonely now that they had been when they were younger, and talked of becoming increasingly lonely as time went on.

I feel lonely, oh yes, I think everybody feels lonely sometimes. And then you pull yourself together and you think well it's ridiculous, you know. . . . it's just happened in these last two years really, two or three years. I'm missing him more now, these last three or four years, than I have since he died, you know. Because he died within five minutes, you know, it was all over very quickly. I mean he wasn't ill and I didn't have to look after him or anything. [209: 4: 50]

There was a group of people who categorised themselves as becoming more lonely but suggested that this was a gradual process that occurred over a period of time, caused by a gradual series of losses rather than a single, identifiable event. Contributing factors included friends moving away or dying, changing neighbourhoods, retirement, and children moving away, which resulted, either directly or indirectly, in a reduction in the social interaction available to the person.

> I lived in London all my life and I actually ended up living in the house that my grandmother owned so I had known the property since I was 10. And I didn't know the name of the people that lived opposite me. And the other thing that happened in the East End where I lived, and please don't misinterpret this that I'm racist, because I don't think that I am racist, but it ended up that when I moved out I didn't have one white neighbour. And I felt isolated. And whilst the Indian family that lived next door to me were very nice and very kindly, the women didn't speak English and the only way you could communicate was through the children. . . . you could have no conversation or contact with the women at all. So I did feel totally isolated there. And that was one reason why I moved. Not because they were black but because you couldn't communicate with anybody. It was like living in a foreign country on your own. I lived in a terrace property and the people opposite me, and on both sides, and behind me, were all foreign. So if I had at any time wanted help I would have had to go through the children because they were the only ones that spoke English, and I just felt totally isolated. [305: 4: 32]

> . . . we've got a lot of our friends that have gone abroad to live so they're sort of dwindling. But now we find that as you're getting older you're losing friends. Because we've lost two or three friends that have died recently, you know, and you don't make new ones. I suppose it's because we don't go out. I'm working and we don't go out socially, so you don't really meet new people. [701: 4: 18]

## Consistent and enduring loneliness

Our final group of people were those for whom loneliness was a consistent, constant and enduring experience across the life course. These we termed the 'existential' group and was the least common of the trajectories that we identified in our interviews. This was where loneliness was a constant throughout the life of the person interviewed. Although there were times in their lives where they were more or less lonely, there was always a constant, underlying, theme of loneliness running throughout the life course. Only one of the people that we interviewed could be classified as existentially lonely. She talked about the constant fear of being lonely and the fact that she hated being alone, no matter where, or what time of day or night, or for how long.

Q: So do you ever feel lonely then?

A: Oh yes, even when I'm here. Not so much today, I mean [my friend] has gone out today so I shall go out this afternoon. She's gone to see her daughter. But if I feel that I can't cope then I shall go to bed. It does help me get rid of it ... When I am on my own, if I'm left for say half an hour even, I just go into myself and want to hide. Sometimes I don't want to cope with it at all ... I've never really liked it, even when I was 15 or 16. [102: 6: 44]

This is clearly an extreme example of existential loneliness, where being lonely, and the fear of being lonely, completely take over the life of the participant. It may be that existential loneliness, in a milder form, is more common than people would like to admit, with more people constantly being lonely or fearing loneliness, albeit as a niggling fear rather than a traumatic neurosis. Although it is likely to be quite rare, however, existential loneliness is distinct from the other two types, and needs to be classified in its own right and clearly offers a different type of change in terms of remedial interventions.

These categories were identified from the qualitative analysis. However, by using the responses given in the survey interviews to two questions, current loneliness and changes in loneliness, an estimate of the prevalence of the three categories can be made. Estimating the prevalence of each category within the survey population is dependent upon how the 'intermediate' category of loneliness is handled. Given that we are asking individuals at a single point of time and hence there is no temporal or cultural shift in how they interpret the 'sometimes' lonely category we have used all three categories – always, often and sometimes – in this analysis to determine loneliness. This is an analytical strategy used by others as well; however, we accept that it is problematic.

Using this analytical strategy 76 per cent of survey participants were categorised as experiencing no change in their perception of loneliness; 60 per cent were not currently lonely and had not been lonely previously, whilst 16 per cent were constantly lonely. Nine per cent were defined as 'regenerative' in that their rating of loneliness had improved over time, whilst for 30 per cent it had deteriorated: 22 per cent were 'new onset' and for the remaining eight per cent loneliness had worsened over the decade. So by far the largest group of survey participants with a 'changed' loneliness category were the 'new onset' group and this links to the highly situational or responsiveness nature of much of the loneliness that is observed amongst older people due to bereavement and other losses.

How do the patterns of change in loneliness compare with other studies? Clearly this is problematic because of the very differing approaches used. Dykstra et al. (2006) report that over a 10-year follow-up period the loneliness status of 70 per cent of their participants was unchanged; for 10–13 per cent loneliness decreased whilst for 11–18 per cent it increased. Jylhä (2004) reported that at a 10-year follow-up 51 per cent of participants were not lonely, 13 per cent had improved, 19 per cent were worse and 17 per cent were consistently lonely. Given the different approach used in these studies the patterns of change reported are not dissimilar between the studies.

## Longitudinal studies of loneliness

As we have already noted, it is popularly thought that loneliness is an inevitable experience of later life. We have already demonstrated that loneliness, at least in its most severe form, is a minority experience and this is true for studies undertaken across a broad range of countries and at various time points from the middle of the last century. However, there is a related question and that is: 'Do individuals become lonelier as they grow older?' Clearly our study could not address this on the basis of a single point in time, cross-sectional survey. However, as Dykstra et al. (2006) note, there are very few studies where loneliness is the prime focus of investigation and has been evaluated longitudinally and in relevant study populations using a suitably powered study. Many of the published studies are based upon small sample sizes and/or focus upon specific population sub groups such as university students, widows or men. This is not to belittle these studies. However, it does limit the extent to which we can draw generalisations about the population.

The studies by Dykstra et al. (2006), Jylhä (2004) and Wenger and Burholt (2004) are notable exceptions in that they focus upon the broad population of older people and examine loneliness, and other measures of social exclusion, as their primary 'outcome' variable.

**Table 4.4** Longitudinal studies of loneliness

| Study | Study group | Measure | Follow-up | Place |
|---|---|---|---|---|
| Tijhuis et al. (1999) | 939 men, 65–85 | De Jong (data reported as means) age, period and cohort effects | 5 and 10 years | Holland |
| Holmen and Furukawa (2002) | 1810 people aged 75 | Self-report described changes | 2 follow-ups over 10 years | Sweden |
| Wenger and Burholt (2004) | 534 aged 65+ | Wenger developed typology | 10 and 20 years | North Wales |
| Jylhä (2004) | 1059 aged 60–89 in 1979 | Self-report | 10 and 20 years | Finland |
| Tiikkainen and Heikkinen (2005) | 207 aged 80 in 1990 | Self-report | 5 years | Finland |
| Dykstra (2006) | 3805 aged in 1992 | De Jong index data reported as means | 4 time points over 7 years | Holland |

However, all of these studies have different durations of follow-up, methods of assessing loneliness and depth of other factors that they recorded. Analytical strategies are also different. A summary of six published studies of loneliness and older people is shown in Table 4.4. The recent study by Wilson and colleagues (2007) is excluded from the analysis as the focus of their work is on testing the hypothesis that loneliness is associated with increased risk of Alzheimer's disease whilst the Zutphen study (Tijhuis et al., 1999) only includes men. A key issue for all longitudinal studies is attrition due to death and other reasons. Dykstra and colleagues have complete data on loneliness at each time point for 1701 participants – approximately a third of their initial sample – whilst the paper by Wenger and Burholt is based upon 45 survivors from the 500 participants recruited at baseline 20 years earlier. In varying degrees all of these studies suffer from the attrition of their samples, hence these data relate inevitably to the 'survivors' and this renders them increasingly 'unrepresentative' but no less interesting as time progresses.

In considering the data presented from these studies there are several types of analyses that can be undertaken – all of which offer different (and complementary) perspectives upon loneliness. We can examine

147

**Table 4.5** Prevalence (%) of loneliness at follow-up in different studies

| Study | Baseline | T1 | T2 | T3 |
|---|---|---|---|---|
| Holmen and Furukawa (2002) | 36 | 11 | 13 | 5 |
| Jylhä (2004) | 6 | 4 | 10 | |
| Wenger and Burholt (2004) | 9 | 6 | 9 | |
| Tiikkainen and Heikkinen (2005) | 5 | 8 | | |

the extent of loneliness at 'baseline'; the extent of loneliness at follow-up (these might be multiple follow-ups as in the case of the North Wales Study by Wenger and Burholt (2004)), and changes in perceptions of loneliness at different follow-up points as compared with baseline or earlier follow-up points. Hence, in evaluating these studies, we need to be clear as to what analysis strategy they are following. The variety of methods used to measure loneliness also makes interpretation of results across studies problematic. Over a seven-year period Dykstra and colleagues report increasing loneliness using the de Jong scale from 1.9 to 2.3, but do not present their data in a form which enables us to determine the percentage of their population classified as very lonely. Two of the three longitudinal studies shown in Table 4.5 suggest a pattern of stability in terms of the overall prevalence of loneliness but do not indicate if this is the same group of individuals who have remained lonely at each time point. The analysis is based upon an ever decreasing pool of survivors. It is likely that 'loss to follow-up' via death, non-response, etc. is selective. For example, the South London Health Survey is a two-year follow-up of a cohort of people aged 65 years and over registered with two primary care centres in south London. At baseline there were 1658 participants – two years later this had reduced to 1214 (see Harris et al., 2003). If we examine loss to follow-up by initial loneliness classification differential attrition is observed. Of those at baseline categorised as never lonely, 21 per cent were 'lost' to follow-up compared with 31 per cent of those categorised as sometimes lonely and 43 per cent of those categorised as always or often lonely. There is clear evidence of greater sample attrition amongst those defined as lonely at baseline.

We can illustrate the dynamic nature of loneliness by examining data from three longitudinal surveys and applying a typology of loneliness to them and comparing the results with the ESRC survey. Table 4.6

**Table 4.6** Comparison of changes in loneliness over time (%)

|  | ESRC | Wenger and Burholt (2004) | Jylhä (2004) | Tiikkainen and Heikkinen (2005) |
|---|---|---|---|---|
| Regenerative | 10 | 2 | 7 | 4 |
| Degenerative | 20 | 28 | 25 | 10 |
| Existential | 15 | 17 | 13 | – |
| Never | 55 | 26 | 31 | 85 |
| Fluctuating |  | 28 | 25 |  |

shows that, given the different methods used, the results are remarkably consistent across the studies in terms of the percentages in the
'regenerative' (10%) and 'existential' (15%) categories. Where
the studies do show variability is in the 'never' category, which is much
higher in our study than the longitudinal studies, and the complex
category of those with fluctuating levels of loneliness over time.
However, as the study by Tiikkainen and Heikkinen (2005) illustrates,
studies with small samples are more susceptible to the influence of
small numerical changes on the overall results.

What factors were associated with longitudinal changes in loneliness? Based upon the studies noted above, changes in loneliness
longitudinally were consistently and independently associated with
changes in social ties in terms of both the marital relationship and the
wider social network and health status (see Box 4.1). Other factors such
as admission to care were not consistently measured across studies, so
it is therefore difficult to offer a definitive statement about the
importance of these factors.

The cohort studies based in south London suggest that there may be
differing sets of factors involved depending upon whether we are
looking at loneliness at baseline, predicting loneliness at follow-up
or looking at changes between time points (Victor et al., 2005a).
For predicting changes between baseline and follow-up bereavement
and loss of contact with friends were the most important predictors;
for predicting loneliness at follow-up depression, health rating, time
alone and conflict with family and friends; whilst marital status and
depression were the most important baseline predictors (Victor et al.,
2005a). Clearly there are a number of different ways that we can
categorise changes in loneliness longitudinally and these differences

| Box 4.1 Factors predicting changes in loneliness in longitudinal studies | | |
|---|---|---|
| Jylhä (2004) | Tijhuis et al. (1999) | Holmen and Furukawa (2002) |
| Household size | Change in partner status | Not having a good friend |
| Marital status | Admission to care | Dissatisfaction with relationships |
| Functional ability | Decrease in health rating | |
| Age | | |

seem to be reflected by the involvement of varying 'risk factors'. This again illustrates the complexity of the concept of loneliness and its links into the social environment of older people.

# How does loneliness vary within the older population?

Like many other social phenomena, loneliness is not equally distributed across the older population (see Pinquart and Sorenson, 2001). There are clear 'peer group' related differences in the distribution of loneliness within the older population. The distribution is not random or equal but is associated with specific subgroups or key factors. Like health, income or quality of life there are a multitude of relationships between loneliness and social, material, health and social resources as well as demographic factors. Preliminary analysis revealed that 36 different variables were statistically associated with increased rates of loneliness, many of which have been described in previous studies. Rather than examine each factor individually we first consider these relationships in terms of groups of related factors.

## Loneliness and demographic factors

Research has consistently demonstrated a link between loneliness and a variety of demographic factors including gender, marital status, living alone and age. Consistently research has demonstrated that women report higher rates of loneliness than men. This relationship has remained more or less constant over time and has been observed in a variety of different settings. So in the ESRC survey eight per cent of women and 11 per cent of men reported that they were always or often lonely compared with 10 per cent and 6 per cent respectively by Townsend (1957). Hence it is easy to presume that loneliness in old age is gendered and predominantly a 'women's issue' (see Beal, 2006). The study by Tijhuis et al. (1999) indicates that loneliness is an issue for men and therefore it is far too simplistic to think of loneliness as only an issue for women. As one male participant said:

> You get very lonely because you can't see any purpose. It's the purpose, you need a purpose in life. It's like everything else. Life is in stages, plateaux. You're struggling with exams. Then you're struggling when the results come out. You're elated when you get into university, elated when you get your degree. Then you're on to the next stage. Then you get married. It's important to get married, so that's a plateau. And after two or three years you get a family. Your family is the next plateau. Then you've got a hell of a lot of your life taken up with the children, and partially also to looking after your family as an extension of that, and that's how it is really. [501: 7: 5]

The association with gender is, however, complex as we have discussed in detail elsewhere (Victor et al., 2005c). It is highly possible that there are factors underlying the issue of gender that are confounding the relationship. For example, it is well established that women are older, more physically frail, more likely to be widowed and more likely to live alone than their male counterparts. The relationship between gender and these other confounding factors could be the underlying reason for the observed association between gender and loneliness. Furthermore, we might speculate that men and women might respond to the questions on loneliness differently.

Age, too, is often linked with loneliness. In the ESRC survey the percentage of those reporting that they were often or always lonely rose from six per cent of those aged 65–74 years, to 13 per cent for those aged 75–84 years and 18 per cent for those aged 85 years or over. Several participants thought that there was an important link here as follows:

I could see that I would be lonely and the reasons are obvious really aren't they, because all of your own generation and your friends have probably all passed away or you don't see much of them, and you would probably find difficulty in making friends when you get to that age. So I would imagine that very old people are more likely to be lonely then people who are our age, because nowadays 60 or 70 isn't all that old like it used to be. It used to be three score years and 10 and you've had it but not nowadays. [101: 8: 39–44]

It is generally assumed that living alone is strongly associated with loneliness. At a preliminary level of analysis there are high rates of loneliness amongst those who live alone with 17 per cent of this group reporting that they were often or always lonely compared with two per cent living with others. Of those defined as often or always lonely, 60 per cent lived alone. Similar findings have been reported previously. For example, Bond and Carstairs (1982) report that, of those living alone in their Scottish survey, 15 per cent were often lonely compared with three per cent of those living with others. More recently Savikko et al. (2005) have reported increased rates of loneliness amongst older people in Finland who live alone, as has also been observed in North America, Australia and Taiwan (Yeh and Lo, 2004b). However, we need to be cautious in stressing this relationship. The variable 'living alone' is a classificatory one and, as Sheldon (1948) noted, older people may maintain a dwelling where they nominally reside alone whilst being enmeshed in a complex web of relationships.

In addition we also observed a relationship between being alone and the amount of time that people reported spending alone and reported loneliness. Solitude and spending considerable amounts of time alone are associated with loneliness. Only four per cent of participants reported that they were always alone whilst 31 per cent stated that they were often alone and 65 per cent seldom or never alone. Amongst those who were always or often alone 18 per cent reported that they were often or always lonely compared with one per cent of those never alone. How has this changed over time both for the individuals in the study and when compared with previous cohorts of older people? Compared with 10 years previously, 34 per cent of participants stated that they spent more time alone, 15 per cent spent less time alone and the remainder were unchanged. Again, those who reported that they spent more time alone than in the previous decade had higher reported levels of loneliness: 18 per cent of this group were often or always lonely compared with three per cent of those whose evaluation of the time they spent alone had decreased or remained static.

The relationship between being alone and feeling lonely is clearly complex. Indeed this distinction was drawn by one of our participants and their spouse as follows:

B   Would you want to differentiate between being lonely and being alone? I think you can be alone without being lonely can't you?

C   And you can be lonely with other people.

B   Yes, I suspect it's possible to be lonely in a group, so I think loneliness and being alone are different things.

C   I suppose ultimately we're all alone.

B   Yes, I don't think I've ever actually been lonely though, but I would imagine it's a feeling that no one cares about you, that if you were in a crisis you would have no one to turn to. And that there's no one really close to you. [404: 7: 12–14]

However, being alone and spending time alone is not an exclusively negative experience. In the qualitative interviews we asked people whether they were happy spending time on their own. Eight participants said that they were happy to spend time alone and, if anything, would like to have more time to themselves and 16 participants were happy to sometimes spend time alone. Twenty participants said that they didn't mind being alone although they would prefer to have company, and only one participant said that they hated being alone and were never happy being alone for any length of time.

Regardless of age, bereavement and widowhood have consistently demonstrated significant and stable associations with loneliness (Van Baarsen et al., 1999; McInnis and White, 2001; Van Baarsen, 2002). Similar associations were found in the ESRC survey: 20 per cent of widows and widowers were often or always lonely compared with one per cent of the married participants, nine per cent of the single (never married) participants and 8 per cent of those who were divorced. The loss of a lifelong companion was something that participants in the qualitative interviews spoke about with elegance and deep feeling. For example one participant reported:

Q: So do you ever feel lonely?

A: Sometimes, yes love. Not having anyone here. The wife.

Q: So it's just since your wife died that you've felt like this?

A: Yes. We used to argue like hell, but I did love her. I miss her. [401: 5: 20]

The loss of a spouse or partner reaches into all aspects of life as this interview extract illustrates:

Q: Do you ever feel lonely?

A: Yes at times I do.

Q: Is that only since your husband died?

A: Oh yes definitely, as I say, there are problems that I couldn't talk to my children about. I do feel lonely at times. And it would be lovely to have my husband. When my husband was alive we went out to the ballet or the opera quite frequently up in London. I used to go with my daughter in Scotland before she got married too.

Q: Do you think it all hinges on your husband's death then?

A: Mmmm, yes. You see you have a totally different, suddenly you're in a different world. I'd always got my husband to lean on and suddenly there's nothing there. And you can't prepare yourself for it.

Q: How would you define loneliness then? I mean were you lonely before your husband died?

A: I think it's not having him. I never felt lonely before, never felt that. [703: 6: 32]

However, one participant did draw an interesting and important distinction between loneliness and the feelings of loss resultant from widowhood as follows:

I don't know really, whether it's a temperamental thing. On the other hand, I can understand it's a different kind of loneliness with friends of mine that they've had when their husband or wife has died. I mean that's a different kind of loneliness, it's a great sense of loss. But I don't think if I feel lonely it's a sense of loss. [106: 5: 19–23]

## Loneliness and health

Loneliness is associated with a broad range of physical and mental health problems as well as a range of measures that relate to how participants evaluated their health status and how their health matched their expectations. This link between loneliness and health status is strong and consistent with loneliness linked with mortality, coronary disease, inflammation, chronic diseases and mental well-being (Hawkley et al., 2006; Heinrich and Gullone, 2006; McDade et al., 2006; Tomaka et al., 2006) and health behaviours (Lauder et al., 2006a). In the survey loneliness was elevated amongst those with a range of physical health problems. Of those with a long-standing limiting illness eight per cent were often or always lonely compared with four per cent of those without such problems. Approximately 12 per cent of those with sight and hearing problems reported that they were often or always lonely compared with eight per cent of those without those problems. The link with visual impairment is consistent with the study reported by Verstraten et al. (2005). Loneliness also showed an association with how individuals rated their own health. Of those who thought that their health was worse than they had expected in old age, 15 per cent were often or always lonely compared with eight per cent of those who felt that their health was either the same as or better than expected. Similarly, seven per cent of those who rated their health as good were often or always lonely, nine per cent of those who rated their health as fair and 19 per cent of those who rated it poor. We should also not forget the importance of a spouse or partners health in the development of loneliness:

Q: Does your wife's health affect the way you spend your time?
A: Well, I mean it restricts, I mean I used to go out much more of a night to committee meetings. Now since she's had the angina ... I was advised not to leave her on her own, I have to curtail that, unless my daughter's down. I used to always go up to the sports and social club monthly meetings but I had to stop that. I go out shopping and leave her for half an hour and it's alright but I don't like leaving her at night. [104: 7: 39]

I go and see my wife on Tuesdays after lunch, and I get there at about 2 o'clock. In order to have contact with her, because there are some days she is ... well she's not ... never is she ... I can never hold a conversation with her, because, you know, she doesn't have any short memory, or any sort of memory at all. She'll talk gibberish to me and I'll have to say oh really, fancy, that sort of thing. I can't say, if I say something or ask her a question it doesn't mean anything, she can't take it in. So, to have some sort of contact with her, and I know this might sound odd, but I take ... because I get there at the time when they have their afternoon cup of tea, and they have tea and biscuits in the afternoon, I do a bit of cooking and

155

I take jam tarts and slices of sponge cake which I make. And sitting there with her, facing her, I feed her with these. She can't feed herself. I mean if I were to put something in her hand, a jam tart in her hand, she wouldn't know what to do with it. And I show it to her and she opens her mouth and I feed her, and so on like that. So they have to feed her all the time. So I do that when I go and see my wife. I stay there just over an hour, halfway through she'll sort of look at me and say oh hello. [205: 3: 14]

An important relationship and enduring relationship has been documented between loneliness and mental health. Studies have linked loneliness with poor mental health, especially depression (Alpass and Neville, 2003; Adams et al., 2004; Tiikkainen and Heikkinen, 2005; Cacioppo et al., 2006). In our study we used the General Health Questionnaire (GHQ) (Goldberg and Williams, 1988) – a general indicator of mental well-being. This revealed that 22 per cent of participants were defined as having poor psychological well-being. In addition, eight per cent reported that they had been told by their GP that they had 'depression'. Of those in the survey who reported that they had been treated for depression, 26 per cent reported being often or always lonely compared with two per cent of those without such an experience. There is an obvious and consistent link between loneliness and depression – indeed the CES-D depression index, but not the Geriatric Depression Scale, includes a question about loneliness within it. Hence when studies demonstrate a link between depression and loneliness this is not surprising if both indices contain a measure of 'loneliness'. Depression is a problem that often accompanies loneliness and depressive symptomotology such as withdrawal, anxiety, lack of motivation and sadness mimic and mask the manifestations of loneliness. In such cases, people are often treated for depression without considering the possibility that loneliness may be a contributing and sustaining factor in their condition.

Whilst there is an easy assumption that these two states are synonymous they are, as we have suggested, in fact two distinct but related concepts, as Weiss (1973) pointed out. Many lonely people say they are depressed and many depressed people say they are lonely but, while the two constructs overlap, they are not identical (Russell, 1982; Alpass and Neville, 2003). Weeks et al., (1980) measured 333 people on both depression and loneliness inventories. He reported that while the two were correlated at 0.49, each was also correlated with different factors – depression was correlated with anger and dissatisfaction with non-social aspects of a person's life, while loneliness was associated with impoverished social relations, especially with friends. More specifically we can see that rates of loneliness are higher amongst depressed elders. For example, in the Leiden 85+ survey 55 per cent of those classed as depressed by the GDS reported that they were lonely compared with 12 per cent for the 'non' depressed (Stek et al., 2004). In the ESRC survey 28 per cent of those with a severe GDS score were often or always lonely compared with eight per cent in the intermediate GDS category and four per cent of those with a 'normal' GDS score. However, as these data demonstrate the association between loneliness and depression is far from 'perfect'.

Whilst not articulating a discourse around depression several participants felt that mental well-being was important in the genesis of loneliness as this comment illustrates:

> We don't need to see other people. I would say if you are mentally disturbed, which please God we're not, erm ... if you are mentally disturbed I would think the lack of contact with other people would really play on one, but we are not, fortunately, in that category. But that's how I would put it. If anyone was mentally disturbed and was, say, without a close family, then no doubt it would play on them mentally. [103: 6: 30]

Clearly those who are both lonely and depressed experience both sets of factors but it is evident that these are two distinct but overlapping states with loneliness independently predicting depression, as measured by the GDS. Whilst the GHQ is not a direct measure of depression the relationship with loneliness illustrates this point. In the survey four per cent of participants demonstrated loneliness and psychological distress, four per cent were lonely but not distressed and 16 per cent had a GHQ score indicating psychological morbidity but not loneliness. Hence both theoretically and empirically, although there is some link between these two states, they are distinct states and should be recognised as such.

Cutrona (1982) distinguishes between chronically lonely people and situationally lonely people – those whose loneliness stems from a specific change in their circumstances. We may speculate that it is the former who are most are likely to be depressed as well as lonely while the latter are more likely to be merely lonely. These categories are similar to the distinction between 'late onset' loneliness occurring often in response to a change in life circumstances and loneliness that has been consistent over the life course: existentialist loneliness. These are two quite distinct states, with differing sets of risk factors and which may, potentially, require differing sorts of remedial interventions (Cohen-Mansfield and Parpura-Gill, 2007).

## Loneliness and material resources

We examined the link between loneliness and three rather crude measures of material resources: housing tenure, educational qualifications and access to a car. Previous research has not extensively examined the link between loneliness and material resources although, recently, Cohen-Mansfield and Parpura-Gill (2007) suggested that financial factors were linked with loneliness. All three measures of material resources demonstrated a statistical link with loneliness. Rates of loneliness were higher amongst those who rented their housing compared with home owners (14 per cent compared with eight per cent) and those without education qualifications compared with those with such awards (12 per cent compared with four per cent). Indeed several participants observed the link between loneliness and material resources as follows:

> We get out when we can but we haven't got the money to do as much as we would like. That's why we moved up here. Because when we retired, we retired in 1990, I sold my business and it was let out and they went bust and we've lost all of our extra pension. So we sold our house down there but we haven't got the money we should have had so it means we can only go out sometimes. ... We used to play golf, but I don't think I could now in any case because of the arthritis, but we would have played up here, you know, if we'd come up here before when we'd got the money. And there's a lot of other things we would have joined. We tend to join things that don't cost much. [601: 3: 13]

> I should think another thing is if one's financial circumstances are not very good this must have a bearing on what you can do. Living on a basic pension I think one could find that you're out, your contact with other people is not very good because the basic state pension is very low indeed. [203: 6: 30–3]

There was a very strong association between reported loneliness and access to a car: five per cent of those with a car reported that they were often or always lonely compared with 15 per cent of those without. Clearly it is not necessarily the car itself that appears to confer a reduced risk of loneliness but the potential it offers for social inclusion (Davey, 2007) and, perhaps, as an indirect indicator of wealth and more broadly defined material resources.

> The car is the independence. The car gives me the means of visiting my friends and my family, because my family don't live on my doorstep, they're all around. But my car gives me the independence to go and see them. Everything revolves around the car, my whole lifestyle revolves around the car really. Because if I'm fed up I go out in the car, and if I want to visit family or friends I'm in the car. And the security of the car as well, because I can drive home from where ever I am and it gives you a sense of security. But I would say that is the main thing. If I had to get rid of anything I think the television would go first before anything, but the car is what enables me. [305: 9: 10]

## Loneliness and social resources

In our initial analyses we included a broad range of variables indicative of the social resources available to participants. These included contact with family, friends and neighbours, activities and availability of a confidant. None of the variables recording contact with family, friends and neighbours were linked to loneliness, as was reported by Routasalo et al. (2006) and perhaps this why 'befriending' schemes have limited effectiveness (Andrews et al., 2003; Findlay, 2003). This is at odds with the comments of our qualitative study participants who felt that links with family and friends were the key to the definition and understanding of loneliness, as these comments indicate:

> We've got a lot of our friends that have gone abroad to live so they're sort of dwindling. But now we find that as you're getting older you're losing friends because we've lost two or three friends that have died recently, you know, and you don't make new ones. [701: 4: 18]

> That is a problem because a lot of friends that we've got are beginning to disappear. And I suppose a big problem is when you get a bit older and then most of your friends have died. [201: 3: 46]

> I've got two brothers and I did have two sisters but sadly I lost my eldest sister last year, she died. But I've got a sister in Chattersley which is local. We always kept in touch, we always visited. [405: 2: 3]

A: My sister takes up a lot of my time and of course my grandchildren down in Canterbury ... I've got a brother is Australia ... I've got a sister who lives in Harrow on the Weald ... And then I have another sister who lives in Derbyshire ...

Q: So do you think having a close family helps?

A: It does, yes, I think so. I don't think I'd like it if I rowed with one and I didn't speak to them for ages, you know. [503: 5: 1]

However, it was not simply the quantity of relationships but their quality that was important for our participants as this comment illustrates:

Now you see I say to you that I am lonely. I think many of my friends would be surprised to hear me say that because they think I've got lots of interests. You know I could have a party and invite 50 or 60 people. I have got friends but they are not the quality of friends that I would like to have in just a few friends. [207: 12: 15–19]

The social resource factors statistically associated with loneliness were voting, going outside of the house, engaging in activities and the availability of a supportive relationship. So we see that eight per cent of those who voted in the previous election were often or always lonely compared with 14 per cent of those who did not. Those who did not participate in an activity in the previous week had higher rates of reported loneliness than those who did (seven per cent compared with 18 per cent). The presence of a confiding relationship was associated with markedly lower rates of loneliness: eight per cent of those who had such a relationship reported that they were often or always lonely compared with 21 per cent of those who did not. It was only the latter factor that was evident in both the survey data and the qualitative interviews. The loss of such a relationship could be devastating as this quote illustrates:

Q: So do you have a close friend that you can talk to?

A: You see, I did. But that's the one who died earlier this year, and I am missing her very much. [207: 8: 4]

## Loneliness – identifying risk and protective factors

We have already indicated that there are inherent limitations to the analysis of individual relationships and the extent of loneliness because

**Table 4.7** Factors associated with loneliness in multivariate statistical models: cross-sectional studies only

| Factor | Victor et al. (2005) | Savikko et al. (2005) | Wenger self-assessed (1996) | Wenger composite (1996) | Jylhä (2004) | Routasalo et al. (2006) | Hall and Havens (1999) |
|---|---|---|---|---|---|---|---|
| Widowhood/marital status | + | + | + | | + | + | + |
| Low income/educational qualifications | ?* | + | | | | | |
| Poor functional status/ disability/restricted mobility | | + | + | + | | + | |
| Living alone/household composition | | + | + | + | + | + | + |
| Self-assessed health/poor health rating | + | + | + | + | | + | + |
| Female | | + | | | | | |
| GHQ/mental health poor/ morale | + | | + | + | | | |
| Expected health in old age | + | | | | | | |
| Time alone | + | | | | | | |
| Increased loneliness over last decade | + | | | | | | |
| Increased age | + | | | | | | |
| Socially active | | | | | + | | |
| Living in an institution | | | | | + | | |
| Depression | | | | | | + | |
| Unfulfilled expectations of contact with friends | | | | | | + | |
| Unfulfilled expectations of contact with grandchildren | | | | | | + | |
| Unfulfilled expectations of contact with children | | | | | | + | |
| 'Poor understanding by close people' | | | | | | + | |
| Low number of contacts | | | | | | | + |
| High number of chronic illnesses | | | | | | | + |
| Local friends | | | + | + | | | |
| Network type | | | | + | | | |
| Time known confidant | | | | + | | | |

161

of the inter-relationship of factors such as age, gender, marital status and living alone. Whilst it is a useful and informative exercise to look at factors individually it is inevitably flawed because of the issue of confounding. However, employment of statistical techniques can help us identify the independent significant statistical relationships. Using logistic regression modelling indicated that there were a set of factors associated with loneliness. These included marital status (widowhood), education (low educational qualifications), poor self-rated health, poor mental health and expectations of health in old age (see Table 4.7). The association of these variables with loneliness perhaps reflects the essentially self-referential nature of the experience of loneliness. Loneliness reflects how we feel about the quality and quantity of our social relationships. This perhaps explains the links with expectations about other spheres of life in old age such as health and self-rated health.

Our analysis demonstrated that certain long-established relationships were not maintained, such as age, gender and living alone. This challenges some very strongly held beliefs about loneliness and its distribution within the older population. Whilst our analysis is not definitive it suggests that it is worth revisiting old preconceptions and subjecting them to rigorous examination.

We have argued that, on the basis of our data, the key factor underpinning the link between loneliness and gender is widowhood (Victor et al., 2005c). Certainly both our quantitative and qualitative studies emphasise the importance and primacy of the marital relationship, as these comments indicate:

> But the only thing is we don't get lonely because we've got each other. [they hold hands] If we were alone, either one of us, I think we would be very lonely because there would be no ... [103: 6: 36]

> I'm bound to feel lonely, I mean having been married all those years. [205: 5: 36]

> I think it's not having him, I never felt lonely before, never felt that. [301: 6: 42]

Similarly the long-established relationship between loneliness and living alone was no longer significant once other factors such as age and marital status are taken into account. This challenges the easy presumption that increased levels of solo living across the age neces-sarily implies a rise in loneliness or isolation or both since neither was linked to living alone once other factors were taken into account. This refutes a very commonly held stereotype that living alone in later life inevitably brings loneliness and isolation and that living alone is implicitly an index for social breakdown and neglect. Clearly our analysis suggests that living alone is simply a summary of the type of household in which an individual lives and does not imply anything about people's social arrangements. Sheldon cast doubt upon the value of the category 'living alone' as an indicator of older people's social contacts when he noted 'the extent to which old people who are ostensibly living alone – and would be so recorded in a census of domestic state – are in actual fact by no means living alone, but are in close and regular contact with their children' (Sheldon, 1948: 140).

There are comparatively few studies that have undertaken multi-variate statistical analyses of the predictors of loneliness in the general population of older people, largely because of the recency of the availability of statistical software and powerful computing facilities. As Table 4.7 shows there is some consistency across studies in highlighting the importance of health experience and widowhood and material circumstances. The situation for other factors remains inconsistent and probably reflects the differing combination of measures included across studies and the sample sizes and varying types of statistical modelling used.

## Conclusion: older people's perspectives on loneliness

In this chapter we have looked at the statistical links between reported loneliness and a variety of key health, social and demographic factors. Such associations are informative and help to us identify those groups within the population most at risk of experiencing this condition. Collation of data across studies strengthens the robustness of our conclusions. However, this does not provide much in the way of developing our understanding of what older people think causes loneliness and how they understand the concept. Indeed, there are few such studies available which look explicitly at the older person's per-spective of loneliness (McInnis and White, 2001) and exclusion (Scharf et al., 2005b), although such perspectives are implicit in the work of Phillipson et al. (2001) and Townsend (1957) and there is some work from the service providers' perspective (Russell and Schofield, 1999). In this section we consider firstly how older people understand lone- liness and then consider what they think places them at risk of experiencing this state. Whilst we separated out these two aspects of loneliness our participants did not always differentiate between the definition, causes or consequences of loneliness nor between loneliness and isolation. However, as several participants commented, this was a hard concept to define:

> I don't know, I really don't know. This is one of the things why I said I didn't think I'd be able to help you. Because I don't think I know enough about loneliness. [404: 7: 2–14]

> Erm … gosh that is a difficult question. [602: 5: 45–6]

Nevertheless we asked participants to describe for us what they thought loneliness was. Overwhelmingly our participants defined loneliness in terms of an absence of social networks and relationships. This was linked to the idea that loneliness was a feature of the number of friends and relations that you have around you and the closeness of the relationships that you have with these people. This is very much in common with the view, reflected in the literature on loneliness, that loneliness is caused by an inadequate social network. Twenty of the people that we interviewed stated that a person's social network is the single most important thing when looking at whether or not a person is, or is going to become, lonely. For the majority of the par- ticipants the most important aspect of the social network was the presence or absence of a partner or confidante. As we have already seen the analysis of the survey data pointed toward the importance of the absence of a partner or confidante as a key risk factor for loneliness. These comments illustrate the varying dimensions of this risk factor for participants:

> Loneliness … It can be almost physical … I've got everything but I haven't got enough. I … er … you can never replace a wife. You can never replace a partner. You can't turn it on and off like a tap. If you love somebody for that many years, it's a very lonely life. [402: 5: 25]

Well before I went into hospital for this hip operation I knew I'd got trouble with my CD-ROM. So I asked one of the men at the group and he tried to tell me but I couldn't work out what to do. Well I had been worrying about this for weeks and the technician at the adult education place came out and had a look at it. He spent three hours on Saturday afternoon doing it for me. Well I haven't really had a chance to play with it yet. Now you see when Joan phoned me on Sunday morning quite early if she'd said anything about how are you or what are you doing, I was so thrilled to bits that this chap had just mended my computer I would have been very pleased to tell her. She never asked so she doesn't know. That's the sort of thing. I don't know If I'm explaining it very well. You hear an awful lot from Help the Aged about poor old souls in unheated rooms and that sort of thing, I think they're lonely because no one ever speaks to them. I'm not lonely in that sense, and I'm not lonely in the material sense because if I want something I could go out and buy it but it's a different kind of loneliness. [207: 22–30]

I would define loneliness I think as if I didn't speak to anybody for a whole day. And I was indoors or didn't see anybody for a whole day. I'm fortunate in as much as I've got the phone and if I want to I can ring up and have a chat with somebody. I think loneliness would be the lack of human contact. I think that's how I would define loneliness. I think a lot of people feel that gap by having an animal, a cat or a dog or something like that. But a cat or a dog wouldn't fit in with my lifestyle. Perhaps if I didn't have the car and I couldn't get out and about it will be a different thing. But I think the lack of human contact would be my deciding factor in loneliness. [305: 6: 43–51]

Another, but rarer, definition of loneliness was articulated in terms of the 'attitude' or psychological disposition of individuals including the ability to find ways of filling time, happiness at spending time alone, the willingness to get up and make yourself do something and the attitude of mind that allows you to go out and meet new people and make new friends, as these comments illustrate:

I think it's an attitude of mind to a great degree. I'm sure there are some really lonely people who really can't help it because of their circumstance, maybe they're unable to get out. I can't understand how people don't have friends, I can't understand anybody not having a friend in the world. But I'm sure there are people who don't. I think it's the attitude of mind of not thinking yourself old. I do not feel old. I still feel in my head

25 or 30, I can't believe it sometimes when I think God I'm nearly 67. It seemed impossible somehow so I think it is partly that if you think old you become old. My sister who is younger than me and has not had a happy life, when she was 60 rang up and said I'm an old age pensioner. And I said no you're not you're 60 years old. And you are not old. It's just your next birthday and you must not think of yourself as a pensioner, you think of yourself as a person who's reached a certain age. She looks much older than me, much older than me, other people have said how much older she looks. And I think it is partly the way she lives and partly her attitude to being old. [502: 5: 37–50]

Well I think it's because we're still looking forward and looking at things to do and places to go, rather than looking back. I think you've got to keep looking forward. But it's not a thing you have to concentrate on doing, it's just your lifestyle isn't it? [702: 6: 29–32]

I don't know really, whether it's a temperamental thing. [106: 5: 23]

I don't think there's any real excuse for loneliness, it might be harder for some people than others to get out, not to feel lonely, but if you make an effort it's not necessary . . . It's just that there are so many things today to help people, to bring them out, to get them to mix with others. I mean there are so many things, there are so many voluntary things that you can join, you don't have to sit back bemoaning your fate and feeling lonely. I'd assume a lot of it is self-induced, surely? [304: 9: 10]

Yes, in similar circumstances, who are single and are just busy all the time and never have time to be lonely. And I think perhaps it is something which you can't quantify because it is something which is within oneself perhaps. One's outlook on life . . . [103: 8: 24–6]

Our participants identified 27 factors as influential when talking about either the causation or prevention of loneliness. These largely followed the typology noted above and focused on social relationships and links with family, friends and the wider community plus specific functional aspects of life such as financial circumstances, health, health of partner or transport that were noted in our initial analysis. These factors are not dissimilar to those reported by Savikko et al. (2005) who asked lonely participants to offer a 'cause' for their loneliness. Illness, widowhood and lack of friends dominated the list, which is remarkably similar to the thoughts of our participants not all of whom were lonely. Again the importance of the partner was paramount:

Are me and my wife happy? You never asked that. And we are very happy. With each other ... it makes an enormous difference. It would be lonely if you didn't talk. [506: 6: 27]

By drawing these strands together we can see a link between loneliness and very close loss, which was identified as a clear causal factor in participant reports of their experiences, or observation, of loneliness. Loss can be separated into two categories dependent on whether they directly or indirectly effect an individual's levels of social interaction. At the most obvious level there is the loss of a partner, confidante, child or best friend, all of which result in the direct reduction of social interaction through the loss of contact with that individual. In addition, there are the losses which indirectly affect levels of social interaction. These include the loss of health, mobility, financial independence, transport and paid employment and the change in the nature of the external environment or neighbourhood. These losses indirectly affect the individual's propensity to loneliness through the restriction of their means of accessing social interaction. We return to these points in Chapter 6.

# 5

# Social exclusion and social isolation

In Chapter 2 we examined the theoretical and conceptual foundation of two of the key concepts in studying the social world of older people: isolation and loneliness. These remain an important part of contemporary debate about quality of life in old age and the degree of social involvement of older people within contemporary society (Barnes et al., 2006). These concepts link to a key element of contemporary social policy thinking concerning the promotion of quality of life in old age through social engagement and social inclusion (Office of the Deputy Prime Minister, 2006; WHO, 2002). In this chapter we provide a brief overview of the concepts of social exclusion and social inclusion and their relationships to social networks as a prelude to examining the degree of 'social exclusion' and 'social inclusion' within our study group. Whilst the focus inevitably is drawn to ideas of exclusion and isolation we seek to foster a sense of perspective by looking at the included and engaged. We also consider how the nature and use of these concepts have changed over time.

## Social exclusion and social inclusion in later life

The interest in social exclusion and social inclusion in later life has not developed in a vacuum. Rather it reflects a wider policy agenda concerned with enhancing 'social inclusion' across society and with enhancing social cohesion by strengthening social engagement: a policy initially articulated with specific reference to young people and with a very heavy focus upon employment opportunities. This concern developed across Europe in response to the perception that the traditional approach to social inclusion, via labour market participation as a means of accessing social rights, was seen to be failing or at least under pressure.

However, the idea of 'social inclusion' translates into policies aimed specifically at older people. The key policy objective for older people since the 1950s has focused, in various guises, on the maintenance and enhancement of quality of life. This is illustrated by policy documents developed at national levels such as the Strategy for Older People in Wales produced by the National assembly (http://new.wales.gov.uk/topics/olderpeople/?lang=en); Opportunity Age – the UK strategy (http://www.dwp.gov.uk/opportunity_age/) and international documents such as the WHO statement on active ageing (WHO, 2002). Manipulation of the social environment by, for example, interventions to promote social engagement and combat loneliness and isolation may offer pathways for the achievement of this policy goal (Findlay, 2003; Cattan et al., 2005a). Consequently, there is a concern to promote social engagement amongst older people that is manifest in local, national and international policy-makers' increasing interest in social exclusion and social inclusion.

What do policy-makers and academics mean by terms such as social exclusion or social inclusion? Like the concept of 'community care', notions of social exclusion and social inclusion manifest many different conceptualisations with a variety of different terms and concepts being used interchangeably (Scharf et al., 2001 and 2002). An essential facet of the idea of social exclusion is the breakdown of the relationship between individuals and society (Barnes et al., 2006). This is reflected in the focus of the debate on the concerns of younger people and their engagement with the labour market and wider ideas of social and civic participation. For older people the implicit issue of policy concern when discussing 'exclusion' is ensuring that family ties are sustained in order to ensure the continued 'supply' of informal carers to facilitate the maintenance of older people independently at home.

It is not necessary here to provide a detailed overview of social exclusion. However, it is important to note that it has always been a multidimensional concept with links to ideas about economic exclusion (poverty), lack of access to public/state institutions, social participation, spatial segregation and cultural exclusion. These dimensions of exclusion are reinforcing and operate in a multiplicative fashion to marginalise some groups from the mainstream of society. For older people this model is especially appropriate as it is well established that the cumulative operation of disadvantages in terms of health and access to other resources such as finances or care services can interact to reduce autonomy and independence.

Scharf and Smith (2004) have developed a five-fold typology of social exclusion, based upon their work with older people in deprived areas, consisting of the following dimensions:

◆ Exclusion from basic services

◆ Exclusion from social relationships

◆ Exclusion from civic activities

◆ Exclusion from material resources

◆ Neighbourhood exclusion

These dimensions form the framework used in the English Long-itudinal Study of Ageing (ELSA) (Barnes et al., 2006). Clearly two dimensions, civic engagement and social engagement, are strongly linked to the concerns of this book and we have examined these individually in Chapter 3. Not all aspects of this model of social exclusion were included in our study and so we cannot examine the distribution and nature of social exclusion within our population. However, secondary analysis of the data from ELSA revealed that, for the population of Britain aged 50 years or over, 29 per cent were excluded on one dimension, 13 per cent on two dimensions and seven per cent on three or more dimensions – this later group defined as being multiply excluded (Barnes et al., 2006). Overall Barnes et al. (2006) report that exclusion from social resources was reported by 12 per cent of those aged 50 years or over, ranging from nine per cent of those aged 50–59 to 25 per cent of those aged 80 years or over. The reality of such exclusion and the impact it has on the daily lives of older people is vividly described in the interviews and case studies reported by Scharf et al. (2005a).

In this chapter we are focusing upon those who are excluded in terms of levels of overall social participation rather than socially excluded per se. However, we acknowledge that this is one very important element of notions of social exclusion. Additionally we shall link our analysis to the dimensions of exclusion proposed by Scharf and Smith (2004) as appropriate even though our study may not have directly focused upon specific aspects of the model such as material resources or access to services.

## Social engagement

Social engagement is a broad and diverse concept with different sub-divisions relating to notions such as social capital, social participation as measured by activity and contact rates and social networks. Social capital includes notions such as neighbourhood attachment, support networks, feelings of trust and reciprocity, local engagement, personal attachment to the area, feelings about safety and proactivity in the social context network. Social networks include notions of exchange relationships, intimate ties, roles and relationships (see Phillipson et al., 2004).

Within this book we focus upon social contact and social participation, rather than detailed social network analysis. Having established the broad policy context we now examine the concept of social networks and the link with social isolation and engagement and loneliness.

### Social networks

A key element of the debate on social engagement and social participation is concerned with social networks and our interests in isolation and loneliness are clearly linked to this research tradition. Social networks, as broadly defined, describe the web of social relationships within which individuals are located. This is a key social science concept with a long historical pedigree that derives originally from social anthropology and is one where sociological perspectives have also been important (see Phillipson (1997) for a review of the sociological contribution to understanding social relationships in later life). Recently there has been considerable energy expended upon developing measures and typologies of social networks appropriate for use with older people (Wenger and Jefferys, 1989; Lubben et al., 2006).

Various authors including Bowling et al. (1989) have clarified the distinctions between social network and social support and, more specifically, between instrumental and emotional support (see Seeman and Berkman, 1988). A social network is the set of people with whom one is in contact and with whom one has some form of social bond. Research has predominantly focused on documenting the structural elements of networks (numbers of contacts, etc.) rather than the 'functioning' of networks. Social support refers to the process by which emotional, financial or physical (instrumental) help is accessed from the network. Social support can then be conceptualised as the social network mobilised to respond to a need for help of some kind by a network member. However, our evidence base as to how support is accessed and mobilised is slim – research has focused much more on the taxonomic aspects of these social phenomena. Social network research, within the gerontological context, has been important for the way that it has challenged the presumption that 'only' family members are significant in the lives of older people. Such research has also demonstrated how different network members provide various types of support in differing situations: there is a 'specialisation' of support functions. Treacy et al. (2005) report that, despite variations in how networks are conceptualised and measured, international research has consistently demonstrated that the 'social network' of an older person typically consists of six to ten individuals. It is a key assumption of contemporary policy debates that older people, and indeed other groups, wish to extend their social networks. The empirical evidence upon which this presumption is based is flimsy.

In our study we were trying both to establish the broad extent of the involvement of older people in exchange relationships with others – who could they turn to for practical help in a crisis – and the more subjective idea of to whom within their network, if anyone, they felt 'close' or 'intimate' with. We described these data in detail in Chapter 3 and demonstrated that most older people are linked within a web of supportive relationships across and between generations. Most older people, approximately 95 per cent, across Europe are able to identify a 'confidante' with whom they have a close relationship. In the UK and Europe the work of Claire Wenger in North Wales has been highly influential in both drawing attention to the importance for older people of social networks and in collecting meticulous empirical data for the development of a typology of social support networks (see Box 5.1). The importance of this work merits some consideration of the applicability of this typology to populations of elders outside of rural North Wales. Whilst we did not design our study to test the typology

---

**Box 5.1 Wenger's typology of social networks**

*The local family-dependent support network* has a primary focus on close local family ties with few peripheral friends or neighbours. It is often based on a shared household with, or near to, an adult child, often a daughter. Community involvement is generally low. Nearly all support needs are met by relatives. These networks tend to be small and the older person (ego) is more likely to be in less good health than those in other network types.

*The locally integrated support network* includes close relationships with local family, friends and neighbours (who may also be friends). This network type is usually based on long-standing residence and includes active involvement with religious or voluntary organisations in the present or recent past. These networks tend to be larger than other network types.

*The local self-contained support network* typically has arms-length relationships or infrequent contact with at least one relative living in the adjacent neighbourhood, often a sibling, niece or nephew rather than an adult child. Childlessness is common and therefore there is increased reliance on neighbours. Ego is more likely in this network type to adopt a household focused lifestyle with limited community involvement. Networks tend to be smaller than other types.

*The wider community focused support network* is associated with active relationships with geographically distant relatives. Absence of local kin with high salience of friends and neighbours is typical. Ego is generally involved in community or voluntary organisations. This network type is frequently associated with retirement migration and networks tend to be larger than average.

*The private restricted support network* is typically associated with the absence of local kin (with the exception of spouse or partner). Contact with neighbours is minimal and ego will have few friends living nearby or be actively involved in community or voluntary organisations. This network type includes both independent couples and people living alone who are in need of support and have withdrawn or have become isolated from local involvement. Networks are smaller than average.

---

or provide an evaluation of its utility nationally it is relevant to consider the typology within the confines of a national survey and as a context for our later comments about isolation.

The data for the network typology consists of eight questions (see

**Table 5.1** Distribution of network types (5)

| | Ireland[3] | Liverpool[1] | North Wales[1] | Belfast[2] |
|---|---|---|---|---|
| | % | % | % | % |
| Family dependent | 7 | 22 | 15 | 47 |
| Locally integrated | 73 | 46 | 45 | 44 |
| Locally self-contained | 2 | 11 | 9 | 0 |
| Wider community focused | 5 | 4 | 20 | 2 |
| Private/restricted | 2 | 12 | 7 | 6 |
| Inconclusive | 10 | 5 | 5 | – |

Sources: 1. Wenger (1995)
2. Wenger and St Leger (1992)
3. Treacy et al. (2005)
Note: Percentages may not sum to 100% due to rounding.

Table 5.1) divided into three sections: proximity of nearest relatives; frequency of contact with family, friends and neighbours; and engagement in civic activities – in this case, church and other groups. Consequently, the network typology highlights spatial isolation, social isolation and exclusion from community and civic activities, anticipating some of the key dimensions in the continuing social exclusion debate. We observe the cultural and temporal specificity of the area where this measure was developed – rural North Wales with a higher than average level of church attendance. Our study did not precisely replicate all the questions used to derive the typology but we are able to populate with data for the majority of the questions. The majority of our participants were involved with family and friends as we illustrated in Chapter 3 but the lack of specific population norms makes it difficult to put the responses of our participants into context.

Whilst it is not the objective of our study to either replicate the typology or offer a critique there are several pertinent observations that we can make. First, there is a focus upon direct contact that replicates the types of presumptions underpinning social isolation measures. The temporal and spatial context underpinning the development of this measure – rural North Wales in the late 1970s – was a community based upon direct contacts, with a strong tradition of church and chapel attendance and a high proportion of first-language Welsh speakers. However, as we saw in Chapter 3 many contemporary contacts between older people and their families are made by telephone and, in the future, we may speculate by computer and web-based technologies. The value and meaning to older people was not perceived to be diminished by the indirect nature of the communication. Furthermore, the focus in the typology is very informed by the importance of 'chapel' to the support networks of older people. In our study we had to broaden the nature of the question to include the array of faith groups that characterise contemporary Britain. However, as we have already noted, the context where this measure was generated was an especially religious area and the importance of religion does not now necessarily translate to the generality of the contemporary cohort of older people. Indeed we now live in a multicultural society and we need to embrace other faith communities. However, as Chapter 3 revealed, in our study for those who attend faith-based activities these are highly valued – but this was only a minority of older people. For the majority of older people church is not an important element of their social world and this seems to have been true of studies conducted outside of North Wales more generally. The importance of the cultural context within which this measure is used is illustrated by a study from Ireland (Treacy et al., 2005) which reported that 85 per cent of study participants attended church regularly and a further four per cent occasionally. In our study only 29 per cent of participants had been involved in a religious service or faith-based activity in the last month.

How common are the different types of networks defined by the typology? Table 5.1 presents data from a variety of studies, two from rural locations, one from an urban setting and one in a more mixed area and we can see that the typology is dominated by the kin-based forms of network – the dominance of a private, restricted network.

## Social isolation

As we saw in Chapter 2, the term 'social isolation' is widely used but rarely defined. Wenger and Burholt (2004) define this concept as the absence of contact from other people. Developing this further we may distinguish two separate aspects of the concept: isolation of individuals or social groups from wider society and isolation of individuals from primary social groups such as family, friends or neighbours (Tunstall,

1966). Hawthorne (2006) suggests that social isolation has been defined as consisting of some, if not all, of the following attributes:

+ Loneliness

+ Living alone

+ Low levels of social contact

+ Low/no social support

+ Feelings of 'separateness'

+ Isolation/aloneness

These different conceptualisations of isolation are present in the variety of ways that isolation has been defined and measured. There is a clear parallel here with the variety of ways that loneliness has been conceptualised and measured and with the conflation of differing concepts – in this case, the utilisation of living alone or social networks as measures of social isolation. From the perspective of social exclusion the detachment and marginalisation of subgroups within the population has been seen as key. For older people the policy debate, whilst mentioning this, is more concerned with the engagement of older people with family and friends, especially as a way of bolstering support networks. We can see the different conceptualisation of isolation in the indices that have been developed to measure this concept empirically. It is also argued by some that the development of reliable and valid measures of isolation is crucial to both the study of gerontology and the development of appropriate services (Lubben et al., 2006).

Central to notions of isolation has been the idea that the 'absence of contact' from the social context can be quantified and a threshold established below which an individual may be categorised as 'isolated'. As noted earlier, this has parallels with debates about poverty where much energy has been expended upon identifying the point along a continuum of income, expenditure or resources 'poverty' may be defined. Whilst conceptually the notion of isolation can be straight-forward – separation from primary social relationships – operationalising such a concept into a measurable form is more problematic. We may identify two distinct quantitative approaches to the creation of social isolation indices. The first is usually based upon a combination of contact with and availability of family (Kutner et al., 1956; Scharf and Smith, 2004), whilst the second involves the computation of a total 'social contact score' (Townsend, 1957) based solely upon the quantity of contacts within a specified reference period, usually a week. This may be collected either prospectively or retrospectively. For Townsend (1957) in particular isolation was conceptualised very much in terms of social detachment from family and community and was an entity that could be both measured empirically and a threshold established below which isolation existed. Both of these approaches are used in this study, again because we wished to draw comparisons with the work of Townsend (1957) as well as addressing more recent developments in research such as the work of Scharf et al. (2004) in deprived areas that was also funded as part of the ESRC Growing Older programme.

## What is isolation? The older person's perspective

Before examining our quantitative data we should consider how older people understand isolation as opposed to loneliness. There is even less research examining older people's ideas about isolation than there is about loneliness. For our participants isolation was largely conceptualised in terms of geographical distance. For example, one woman reported:

> I feel a bit isolated here and that is one reason why I want to move where there is a bit more going on around me. I mean if I moved to somewhere else where I could take a walk into the town or into the shops or go somewhere and have a cup of coffee. You can't do that here you see, it's a village, and that's another reason for thinking, well, I mean I know I can get in the car and go but you don't always want to bother getting in the car to go out. And also there's the cost of running a car. I mean I'm thinking of moving so I don't have to have a car. The money that I don't spend on the car will be more than enough to spend on taxis to get me where I want to go. In Ipswich I would be able to afford to take taxis and things and I wouldn't have the bother of a car. A car's expensive for one person. [301: 7: 1]

Another described social isolation as a result of social and cultural changes within their immediate environment. Again, as with the previous example, isolation is conceptualised as having a strong spatial or neighbourhood component.

I lived in London all my life and I actually ended up living in the house that my grandmother owned so I had known the property since I was 10. And I didn't know the name of the people that lived opposite me. And the other thing that happened in the East End where I lived, and please don't misinterpret this that I'm racist, because I don't think that I am racist, but it ended up that when I moved out I didn't have one white neighbour. And I felt isolated. And whilst the Indian family that lived next door to me were very nice and very kindly, the women didn't speak English and the only way you could communicate was through the children. ... you could have no conversation or contact with the women at all. So I did feel totally isolated there. And that was one reason why I moved. Not because they were black but because you couldn't communicate with anybody. It was like living in a foreign country on your own. I lived in a terrace property and the people opposite me, and on both sides, and behind me, were all foreign. So if I had at any time wanted help I would have had to go through the children because they were the only ones that spoke English, and I just felt totally isolated. [305: 4: 32]

However, overall, participants found it much more difficult to articulate clear definitions of isolation. This was in stark contrast to the eloquent comments on the nature and causes of loneliness described in Chapter 4. It also mirrors the academic literature where robust conceptual and empirical formulations of the concept of isolation are much less well developed that related concepts such as social support or social networks. However, isolation (Holley, 2007) and loneliness (Murphy, 2006) are both seen to be important in the clinical context as well as for older people living in the community.

## Measurement of social isolation

There are two common approaches to measuring social isolation: the counting of contacts for a defined period and the calculation of 'indices' of isolation based upon a combination of measures related to social contacts, availability of family/friends and, variably, aspects of social support.

### Social contact scores

In calculating a 'social contact' score we can tally for each person their total number of social contacts over a specified period – usually a week.

The work of Townsend (1957) exemplified this approach. He enumerated for his participants the total face-to-face contacts of 10 minutes or more duration during the previous week. Clearly when this method was developed contemporary methods of communicating by phone or email were either not available or not widely available. These measures make no comment upon the quality or emotional context of the interactions. It is a simple tallying of interactions. Having calculated the scores for individuals as a continuous variable an arbitrary cut-off point is determined based on the normative assumptions of the researcher or policy-maker about the nature of isolation in later life. The approach is analogous to the way that poverty has been defined over the past 50 years. This essentially creates a dichotomy – all those below the defined threshold are 'isolated' whilst those above it are not. As with any continuous distribution of scores, where the 'case definition' boundary is drawn is of crucial importance in determining the classification of the population into 'isolated' and 'not isolated'.

In order to facilitate historical comparison we generated a social contact score that was based on data about direct face-to-face social contacts over a week-long reference period. In the survey people were asked to report how often they had seen specific groups of people. From their answers we computed a 'total' direct social contact score that excluded other forms of contact such as phone and email. This approach made direct comparison with previous studies possible. Unlike Townsend's original index (Townsend, 1957) there was no requirement for the social contacts on which the score is derived to demonstrate a minimum duration and we have not included contacts with other residents in the household or contact with service providers or public officials.

The distribution of survey participants' weekly contact scores are shown in Figure 5.1. Face-to-face direct contact and all contacts are shown separately. How does the experience of older people at the beginning of the twenty-first century compare with older people living 50 years earlier reported by Townsend (1957) and Tunstall (1966)? In 2000–1 direct weekly contacts varied from 0 to 15 (mean of 9) and total contacts ranged from 0 to 35 (mean of 15). This is clearly very different from the range of 0 to 51+ reported by Tunstall (1966) and the 2 to 208 reported by Townsend (1957) but perhaps rather more in line with the 0 to 21+ reported in the work of Bond and Carstairs (1982). For the

179

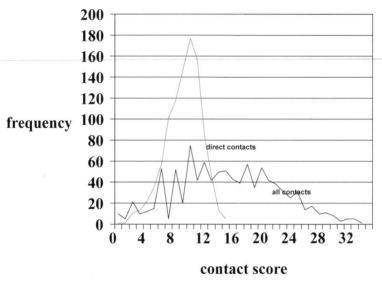

**Figure 5.1** Total weekly contacts

Townsend population the average number of social contacts was 61 per week (median of 52). Both Townsend and Tunstall defined less than 21 contacts per week as indicating isolation. It is not clear as to why this value was selected. Application of this value to our study would result in 79 per cent of older people being labelled as isolated!

Clearly our study has not included all the differing types of contacts that were included by Townsend (1957) and Tunstall (1966). We have included only direct contacts with family, friends and neighbours while they included other forms of contacts such as participation in formal activities. Our study is also retrospective in that participants were recalling contacts rather than recording them prospectively. We also did not apply 'correction factors' to the reported contacts based upon household composition. Although this is a useful mechanism for summarising the variability of older people's social contacts, using this as a mechanism for determining social inclusion or exclusion is problematic because of the essentially arbitrary decision of the cut-off between isolation and non-isolation and the way that the data have been collected. Furthermore, the variations in the data collected across studies makes comparisons of absolute values problematic. It is probably because of these conceptual and measurement issues, especially the definition of what is a social contact, that has resulted in the decline in the use of this type of measure in large-scale surveys. Until the recent interest taken in the area of isolation and exclusion by Scharf et al. (2001) there have been more studies focusing on loneliness rather than isolation. Where isolation is reported it is often via indirect methods such as Tracey (2005) using the Wenger (1989) network typology to impute isolation; via the use of more numerically-based network analyses where the average (mean) number of contacts are computed for differing subgroups but no attempt is made to define a threshold (see Boldy et al., 2004); or via a conflation with loneliness.

Given the conceptual and measurement issues can we draw any comparisons across studies in the classification of participants as isolated? Defining categories of 'isolated', 'intermediate' and 'not isolated' is problematic. Whilst Townsend (1957) and Tunstall (1966) use absolute values to define their groups they do not offer any conceptual, theoretical or statistical rationale for the category boundaries. In this study we have used a set of pragmatic principles based on common sense to determine the limits of isolation and engagement as we are predominantly interested in determining the 'extremes' of our distribution. We have defined isolation as less than one contact per day (i.e. seven direct or phone contacts or less per week) and high engagement as three or more direct or phone contacts a day (a total of 21 or more contacts). The remaining group were defined as 'intermediate' and include the bulk of participants. This gives a 'prevalence' of isolation of 13 per cent that is very similar to the 10 per cent reported by Townsend (1965) but is only half of the 21 per cent reported by Tunstall (see Table 5.2). Bond and Carstairs (1982) do not present their data in comparable terms. However, they report that three per cent of their sample had no contacts in the index week compared with one per cent for our study. Some six per cent of our participants had 1 to 4 contacts and 12 per cent 5 to 9 contacts – compared with eight per cent and 27 per cent respectively in their study. In Wenger's (1984) initial survey in 1979 some six per cent of her sample were defined as very isolated and 26 per cent as moderately isolated. This is about double the level for our study but is based upon a very different type of index. The recent national study of exclusion using secondary analysis of ELSA data reported that 13 per cent of those aged 50 and over were excluded in terms of social participation (Barnes et al., 2006). As with our examination of loneliness, examining cohort-based changes in the prevalence of isolation is problematic because of the variability in the way that isolation is conceptualised and measured and the specificity of the population examined.

We were also interested in the 'engaged'. Using our admittedly pragmatic definition of three or more contacts daily, outside of the household, 23 per cent of participants were highly engaged. Bond and Carstairs (1982) do not present their data in terms of reference to an arbitrary isolation 'cut off'. Rather their data are grouped. In their analysis 26 per cent have 21 or more contacts per week. This group may be taken to be analogous to our 'highly engaged group' who have a similar contact definition threshold. That the size of these two categories is very similar is remarkable given the differing approach used to generate the total contact score. Given the emphasis upon 'active ageing' and 'ageing well' and the emphasis placed upon social engagement as a means of enhancing quality of life these highly engaged elders merit further study. What are their characteristics and how do they differ, if at all, from the general population of older people? We shall return to this point when examining another method of defining the engaged and the isolated.

### Social isolation indices

Composite isolation indices are based upon the presence or absence of particular attributes and a score is calculated for each response – usually on the basis of presence or absence. Some of the widely used or recent indices are summarised in Box 5.2.

Kutner et al.'s (1956) score is based upon five separate variables that are equally weighted and which relate to contacts with key social links, the availability of kinship relationships and the desire and opportunity for making new social links. In Chapter 3 we noted that our participants found making new social links difficult. However, measuring such concepts empirically is problematic. In contrast to the temporally fixed contact scores this measure has a variable timeframe and uses several imprecise concepts such as 'seeing', 'having' or 'making' friends. Empirically this measure is difficult to reproduce because of the imprecise way that the score is computed. Conceptually it is problematic because it links social levels of contact, availability of family and friends and the desire and opportunity for more links within a single measure and attributes equal weight to each dimension.

**Box 5.2 The composition of key social isolation scores**

| Kutner[1] | Wenger and Burholt[2] | Scharf[3] | Scharf[4] |
|---|---|---|---|
| Seeing children monthly | Lives alone | No living children (or child 50+ miles away) | No relatives/ sees them less than weekly |
| Seeing other relatives monthly | Has no close (kinship ties) relatives | No living relatives (or 50+ miles away) | No friends/ chats to them less than weekly |
| Having close living friends | Never visits anyone | Sees child/ relatives less than monthly | Chats to/sees neighbours less than weekly |
| Having personal friends | Has no contact with neighbours | No friends in neighbourhood | |
| Making new friends | Has no telephone | Talks to friends less than monthly | |
| | Is alone for more than 9 hours per day | Talks to neighbours less than monthly | |
| | Nearest neighbour is more than 50 yards away (out of earshot) | Lives alone | |
| | Never goes out of the house | | |

*Sources:* 1. Kutner et al. (1956)
2. Wenger and Burholt (2004)
3. Scharf et al. (2002)
4. Scharf et al. (2004)

In Kutner et al.'s (1956) study 56 per cent of older people were defined as isolated. We cannot replicate this measure for our study as we did not ask about making new friends. Nor did we distinguish between contacts with children and other family members. However, in our study five per cent had no relatives, no close friends or relatives nearby or had not seen relatives in the past month. Additionally, in our study 17 per cent were not in weekly contact with family, friends, neighbours whilst 11 per cent were not in monthly contact. Even given the very different way that we operationalised our measure the levels of isolation are clearly much lower in our study. This undoubtedly reflects the differing nature of the populations included in the studies. It also demonstrates how sensitive estimates of concepts such as social isolation are to the nature of the indices used to construct them.

Wenger and Burholt (2004) report the use of an eight-item isolation score used in the Bangor Longitudinal Studies of Ageing. This is based upon responses to the eight items listed in Box 5.2. This index is very much one that is informed by the socio-cultural context of the study area that it was devised for. As with the network typology several of the items are very specific to the time of the study, for example, phone access and proximity of nearest house. At the time of our study phone ownership was virtually 100 per cent across the population, including older people. Hence we did not attempt to calculate this measure but it is presented so that we can make comparisons with the results of Wenger's very important work.

Recently Scharf et al. (2002) have devised a contemporary isolation index (Scharf index) based upon seven key indicators which they then refined down to three variables related to weekly contact with friends relatives and neighbours. The seven-item index, with a range of 0–7, includes 'living alone', as do many measures, and is seen by Hawthorne (2006) as being a core component of the concept of isolation. However, the inclusion of 'living alone', which is experienced by about a third of our participants, means that the measure lacks precision and focus and identifies a large number of 'false positives'. Indeed in their study of deprived areas only 21 per cent of participants were not defined as isolated using this measure (Scharf et al., 2002).

The revised three-item Scharf index focuses upon contacts only and excludes spatial proximity and household living arrangements. Using this three-item index still only 26 per cent of our participants did not score positively on any of the three items; 49 per cent had a score of 1 (low) whilst two per cent were classified as 'severely' isolated and 23 per cent as moderately isolated. This is a much higher estimate of isolation than reported by Townsend (1957) but is closer to the 21 per cent of Tunstall's (1966) participants that were defined as 'isolated'. Iliffe and colleagues (Iliffe et al., 2007) have used the six-item Lubben Social Network scale to measure isolation amongst older people in London and report a prevalence of 15 per cent. However, this measure includes both levels of contact with family/friends, feelings of closeness with family/friends such that private matters could be discussed with them and sufficient strength of relationship that help could be requested. Clearly this measure is recording isolation plus other aspects of the nature of the relationship between older people and their family/friends.

We can compare, directly, the influence that the two different methods of calculating the score has upon the identified results. Victor and Scharf (2005) report that in the deprived areas 43 per cent were not isolated at all, 37 per cent had a low score, 15 per cent a medium score and five per cent were highly isolated using the three-item index. This contrasts with 26 per cent defined as not isolated, 26 per cent low isolation, 21 per cent medium isolation and 27 per cent high isolation using the seven-item index. Clearly a screening measure or a classificatory tool that only identifies a quarter of the population as 'not isolated' needs further work to make it more precise.

From these comparisons we see considerable variability across studies in the classification of older people in terms of their degree of social isolation. This clearly reflects the differing nature of the methods and measures used to operationalise the concept of isolation. Of particular note is the volatility of the 'intermediate' category reflecting the arbitrary choices of the boundaries drawn between 'not isolated' and 'somewhat' isolated and the nature of the questions used to define the index. Inclusion of living alone as a component of the index inevitably inflates the estimates of isolation. The similarity of the percentage classed as not isolated using our two measures, the contact score and the Scharf three-item index, is notable as is the consistency of the extent of 'severe' isolation at around 5–10 per cent where the measure excludes living alone. Again, as with loneliness, if we exclude measures that include living alone there appears to be a pattern of stability in the extent of severe isolation across the older population (see Table 5.2).

**Table 5.2** Prevalence of social isolation in selected studies

| Study | Measure of isolation | Classification |
| --- | --- | --- |
| Townsend[1] | Weekly social contacts less than 21 = isolated, 22–35 contacts = rather isolated | 10% isolated, 13% rather isolated, 77% not isolated |
| Tunstall[2] | 21 contacts = isolation | 21% isolated, 26% with 40+ contacts per week |
| Wenger[3] | Customised isolation score | 28% moderately isolated, 6% very isolated, 64% not isolated |
| Scharf et al.[4] | 7 item index | 27% highly isolated, 21% moderately isolated, 26% low isolation, 26% not isolated |
| Shanas et al.[5] | Lives alone, no visitors in previous week, no contact in previous day | 2–3% isolated |
| Hawthorne[6] | 6-item friendship index | 4% very isolated, 11% isolated, 17% some isolation, 69% not isolated |
| GO Survey | Social contacts score | 13% less than 7 contacts, 26% over 21 contacts |
| GO Survey | Scharf 3 item index | 2% severely isolated, 23% moderately isolated, 49% low isolation, 26% not isolated |

*Sources:* 1. Townsend (1957)
2. Tunstall (1966)
3. Wenger and Burholt (2004)
4. Scharf et al. (2002)
5. Shanas et al. (1968)
6. Hawthorne (2006)

# Factors associated with social isolation

Is the experience of social isolation equally distributed across the older population? Previous research has suggested that a variety of factors are associated with isolation and these are summarised in Box 5.3. Here we do not list in detail every variable but group them into broad categories. The studies by Townsend (1957) and Tunstall (1966), which provide the context for much of our work, were undertaken when there was only a limited computational capability to undertake statistically based data analysis. Their analysis does not extend beyond the investigation of bivariate relationships using cross-tabulation. Our analyses have demonstrated that there are a variety of different factors associated with isolation. As with our examination of loneliness we first examine the individual associations between isolation and three different factors before reporting multivariate analyses.

Our analysis is complex because of the two different approaches to the measurement of isolation. We first examined the peer group distribution among participants using the contact score as the dependent variable and repeated the analysis using the Scharf index as the dependent variable. However, for the total social contact score

| Box 5.3 Factors associated with social isolation | | |
|---|---|---|
| Demographic factors | Social factors | Health status factors |
| Advanced age | Living arrangement | Self-rated health |
| Gender | Social network | Poor physical health |
| Marital status | Retirement migration | Mental illness |
| Ethnic status | Social class | Admission to long-term care |
| | Intimate social relations | Restricted mobility |
| | Employment status | Limitations in activities of daily living |
| | | Low morale |

the interest was in the links and associations rather than the number of contacts between groups because of the 'indirect' way that the measure had been calculated. For the measures proposed by Scharf there is a further element of complexity and that relates to the number of categories used. Clearly the two indices give each individual a score from 0 to 7 and 0 to 3 respectively. We can probably agree that a score of 0 is clearly indicative of a state of no isolation and a score of 3 or 7 is indicative of isolation but how many categories should we use and where should the boundaries between different categories be drawn? Should we use a two- (not isolated vs isolated), three- (not isolated, intermediate isolation and highly isolated) or four-fold (none, low, medium and high) typology? We examined the relationships using three different formulations of the Scharf index: the detailed four category (grouping the small number of people classed as severely isolated we grouped together the moderate and severe group) and a dichotomy – isolated versus not isolated. Here we were examining two distinct but related questions. Are the patterns of association between isolation and socio-demographic factors constant across the two methods of measuring isolation? Second, does the pattern of association vary with the number of categories of isolation used in the analysis?

In our study there were 31 different variables associated with the social contact measure of isolation (Table 5.3) including demographic characteristics, material resources (car ownership and education), quality of life rating and, not surprisingly, neighbourhood and social resource variables. Many, but not all, of these variables were also associated with loneliness (see Chapter 4).

The largest number of significant statistical associations are demonstrated by the social contact score, whereas the three forms of the Scharf index demonstrate between eight and ten significant statistical associations. Measures of health status, gender and living alone were associated with the social contact score but not associated with any of the variations of the Scharf index. Whilst it is problematic trying to make sense of such a large number of relationships, there are some key issues that are worth focusing on in drawing links with previous studies and with loneliness. Unlike loneliness, there is a strong association between the different indices of isolation and social network variables. The factors identified were broadly stable regardless of

**Table 5.3** Factors associated with the study measures of social isolation – bivariate analysis

| Social contact score univariate analysis | Scharf 2 category score | Scharf 3 category score | Scharf 4 category score |
|---|---|---|---|
| Advanced age | * | * | * |
| Being female | | | |
| Being widowed | * | * | * |
| Living alone | | | |
| Always alone | * | * | * |
| Increased aloneness | | | |
| Contacts with family/friends/neighbours | * | * | * |
| Proximity of family/friends | * | * | * |
| Evaluation of neighbourhood | | | * |
| Availability of help | * | * | * |
| Availability of confidant | * | * | * |
| Knows neighbours | * | * | * |
| Chronic illness | | | |
| Disability | | | |
| Fall in last year | | | |
| Health rated poor | | | |
| Diagnosis of depression | | | |
| GHQ case | | | |
| Sensory impairments | | | |
| Housing tenure | | | |
| Qualifications | | | |
| Access to care | * | | |
| Holiday in last year | | | * |
| Quality of life rating | | | |
| Loneliness | | | |
| Feels safe by day | | | |

the way that isolation was categorised and these broadly mirrored the variables associated with the contact score, with the exception of health status, gender and living alone. However, there is only limited overlap with the factors associated with loneliness. Given the stability of the associations demonstrated across the various ways of categorising the Scharf index we used a three-category measure – severe isolation, low/intermediate (moderate) isolation and not isolated – in reporting the multivariate analyses of isolation.

## Isolation and material resources

One strong theme that emerged from both our quantitative and qualitative interviews was the importance of material resources in facilitating social engagement. As with loneliness, access to a car was associated with social isolation as measured by the total contact score and the Scharf index. The mean number of contacts for those with a car was 9.7 compared with 8.2 for those without a car. However, we should interpret these contact levels cautiously because of the nature of their calculation. Rather than view them as 'absolute' figures we present them as indicative of the extent and nature of differences in contact levels across different groups. Similarly, 22 per cent of those with a car were defined as demonstrating high isolation compared with 29 per cent of those without a car. Previous studies, by focusing on health and socio-demographic factors have, perhaps, underestimated the importance of resources, especially money, in enabling older people to be engaged. These extracts from our qualitative interviews with participants highlight the importance of finances in enabling them to engage socially and thus 'prevent' isolation

> I should think another thing is if one's financial circumstances are not very good this must have a bearing on what you can do. Living on a basic pension I think one could find that you're out, your contact with other people is not very good because the basic state pension is very low indeed. [206: 3: 30–3]

> Well, I mean obviously we have to live within our pensions. Therefore if we had fewer financial limitations we would be able to do more ambitious things. [201: 7: 41–2]

Finances and material resources were also important in enabling older people to maintain a car, which was also seen as key to enabling social interaction, as these extracts illustrate:

> The car is the independence. The car gives me the means of visiting my friends and my family, because my family don't live on my doorstep, they're all around. But my car gives me the independence to go and see them. . . . Everything revolves around the car, my whole lifestyle revolves

around the car really. Because if I'm fed up I go out in the car, and if I want to visit family or friends I'm in the car. And the security of the car as well, because I can drive home from where ever I am and it gives you a sense of security. But I would say that is the main thing. If I had to get rid of anything I think the television would go first before anything, but the car is what enables me. [305: 9: 10]

I shall be very sorry when I can no longer drive because that gets me out and about and gives me independence. You don't have to wait for buses, you don't have to ask people for lifts. I mean that is a wonderful thing, to have independence. [303: 6: 37]

Oh I wouldn't want to be without it [car]. It gives me my independence. I know we're on a bus route but it's still a walk that way or up to the end of the avenue, and another thing, I wouldn't go out at night if I didn't have a car. You hear such dreadful things these days. [405: 3: 1]

It was also seen as a way of creating activities and things to do to avoid being bored.

If I find that I'm getting a bit maudlin I get in the car and go out. And this is one advantage of the car. You can always drive somewhere or go to see someone. I've driven down to the sea front before now and gone into a café and had a cup of tea, and invariably someone will come and talk to you. [305: 6: 35]

We would certainly argue that the importance of material resources, difficult though they are to define and measure, has been under-estimated in studies of social isolation and exclusion although their importance is clearly demonstrated in the comments made by older people themselves (Scharf et al., 2005b).

## Isolation and demographic factors

A particular interest of our research was the relationship between isolation and living alone. Average (mean) social contact scores were lower for those who lived alone, at 8.5 per week compared with 9.4 for those who lived with others, excluding contacts within the household. However, there was no significant association using the Scharf index: two per cent of both those living alone and living with others were severely isolated whilst 25 per cent and 24 per cent respectively were categorised as moderately lonely. Again this challenges the notion that there is an inevitable link between living alone, exclusion and isolation.

It has been argued that both isolation and loneliness are women's issues whilst the English Longitudinal Study of Ageing survey suggests a weak association between social exclusion and being male. We have demonstrated that in our study this was not the case for loneliness (Victor et al., 2005c). With regard to isolation two per cent of both men and women were identified as severely isolated whilst 25 per cent of men and 21 per cent of women were moderately isolated. There is certainly a hint here that men are at least as vulnerable, if not more so than women to the experience of isolation. In part this may reflect their lack of friendship networks, as these comments from our interview respondents hint:

> Ironically, although I had lots of friends at work, although most of them were subordinate because I was the director, but I spent a lot of time travelling. I not only had to travel to and from work because I worked in London, and when I worked in the Wirral I spent a lot of time travelling to London, and I was actually commuting from Guildford to the Wirral because all our customers were in London. And at the weekend, as you will probably know, when you spend the week commuting most of your weekend is actually spent trying to catch up with the things that you should have done during the week but didn't have time ... but unless you are a member of a golf club or something like that you just can't make friends. Women do because they are either working locally or they take the children to school. Chaps see people on the train but they get off the train and that's it. [201: 5: 10]

> I mean when a chap leaves work that's his main conversation. I can say that because prior to the bowls I used to be a volunteer for redundant managers, in city management, and I had a lot to do with men who had lost their jobs. They're all the same. They're very short on friends, real friends. Very short indeed. And when they come to the bowls club they come with marvellous ideas, I'm looking forward to this retirement, I've got the garden to do, I've got the painting to do, I'll be fully occupied. But within three months they normally have a chat with me and say, 'Where do you think I can get a part-time job?' That's the general run of most of the people who are, I suppose, in the semi-professional group ... So that's why, after three months, they finally volunteer to get more work. [501: 4: 6]

We would certainly argue that for both isolation and loneliness the problem is not exclusive to either men or women: both are vulnerable to the experience. However, our research base is not sufficiently robust to determine if there are significant variations in how men and women understand and explain aspects of their daily lives.

## Isolation and health status

As with our results for loneliness there was a series of statistical associations between the social contact score and health status. Consistently mean levels of social contact were lower amongst those reporting the presence of chronic illness, a fall in the previous year, problems with activities of daily living, problems with sight/hearing, poor self-rated health and a high GHQ score. However, the Scharf index did not demonstrate these links. This illustrates how we can identify very different patterns of association between dependent and independent variables depending upon how the dependent variable, in this instance isolation, is defined and measured (a continuous measure of social contacts versus a category index).

## Multivariate analysis

However, it is well established that many of these factors are inter-related and we can now undertake statistical analysis that can exclude the influence of confounding and identify the associations between dependent variables such as social contacts, isolation and independent variables such as age, gender or marital status. Again we continue to use the two differing approaches to the measurement of isolation to examine what, if any, differences in patterns of association this generates (see Table 5.4).

In our analysis only a handful of variables demonstrated statistically significant and independent relationships with both social contacts and the Scharf index. Four were related to the availability of a wide social network: relatives living close by, people to turn to in a crisis and knowing few or no neighbours. In addition, widowhood and access to a car were associated as independent predictors of both social contact and the Scharf isolation index. There were no measures of health status included in the final analysis nor variables such as age, gender or living alone. The importance of neighbours and of knowing one's

**Table 5.4** Variables associated with loneliness: multivariate analysis

| Factor | Social contact score | Scharf 3 category score | ELSA social[1] relationships measure | Wenger[2] |
|---|---|---|---|---|
| Being widowed/years widowed | * | * | | * |
| Contacts with family, friends & neighbours | * | * | | |
| Proximity of family/ friends | * | * | | |
| Availability of help in crisis | * | * | | |
| Availability of confidant | * | * | | |
| Knows neighbours | * | * | | |
| Access to car | * | * | | |
| Living alone | | | * | * |
| No partner | | | * | |
| No children/siblings | | | * | |
| Unemployed | | | * | |
| Male | | | * | |
| Depression/morale | | | * | * |
| Poor health | | | * | |
| Advanced age | | | * | |
| Social class | | | | * |
| Network type | | | | * |
| Time known confidant | | | | * |

*Sources:* 1. Barnes et al 2006
2. Wenger et al 1996

neighbours, even if one was not intimately acquainted with them, was very important as is illustrated by the following interview extracts:

> You see I've got next door, the lady over the road, number 50 down the road, they've all got keys so that if I wanted assistance I could sound the alarm and ask them to come and help me, you know. [204: 4: 43]

> The people at this end of the street are all very neighbourly and look after each other. I mean I know one day I didn't take my milk in very early and somebody came across to make sure I was alright. [206: 2: 28]

Q: How long have you lived in this area?

A: ... Since I were about 24.

Q: So you know this area pretty well then?

A: Fairly well yes.

Q: And do you know your neighbours around here?

A: Erm ... well people change. This is a new neighbour [gesturing] but I know this neighbour here. [406: 1: 21]

Q: So what are the neighbours like?

A: Well there's the house opposite, two more just there and another one further up and they don't even say hello. Never said hello since I've been here. In four years. That's how people are today. Because women they always go out to work now. The man next door this way [gestures], he's a retired doctor, he'll chat when I see him, and the people dead opposite me, but none of the others even say hello. It used to be that everybody used to talk to everybody, knew everybody else. They haven't got the time now. [306: 6: 16]

The remaining variables linked to both social contact and the isolation score were the availability of a confidante, access to a car and marital status. Those with a confiding relationship had an average (mean) of 9.15 contacts per week compared with 6.7 for those without such a relationship. Widowhood has both emotional effects upon an individual's evaluation of their social embeddedness, as we described in Chapter 4, and disrupts and dislocates social networks, as this comment from one of our participants clearly demonstrates:

People that we used to be friendly with suddenly seemed to find me a threat when I was on my own, whilst when my husband was around it was OK. But people stopped inviting me to things. Widows are seen to be a threat and I was only invited if there happened to be a single man invited as well. [507: 4: 38]

Relating these results to previous studies is problematic because of the differing analytical strategies used and the varying ways that isolation has been defined which are, perhaps, even more variable than for loneliness. Given this caveat we can draw a broad comparison with the study of exclusion in the English Longitudinal Study of Ageing (ELSA) (Barnes et al., 2006), Scharf et al. and Wenger (see Table 5.5). This exercise reveals that there is absolutely no agreement between the factors identified in our study and those identified in ELSA (Barnes et al., 2006).

## Cohort and longitudinal changes in isolation

How does isolation change over time? Few researchers have investigated this aspect of social relationships in later life from a longitudinal perspective. Wenger's North Wales study offers some insights into this topic. At a crude level, rates of isolation increased both overall and for survivors only. For the overall group the percentage of not isolated decreased from 64 per cent at baseline (1979) to 36 per cent in 1995. However, the severely isolated group remained remarkably stable (6 per cent at baseline and 4 per cent in 1995). For the survivors the not-isolated group decreased from 64 per cent to 38 per cent and the severely isolated group remained stable at nine per cent. So, as with some of the data for loneliness, the change over time is concentrated in the intermediate category rather than the severe group. Hence to some degree these changes may reflect changes in response to one or two questions, thereby moving participants into a different category when there might have been no fundamental change in their social situation. In particular, we might speculate as to how much the change in the percentage categorised as moderately isolated reflects an increase in living alone in this group. Or how much increased rates of telephone ownership prevented an increase in levels of isolation.

As with their work on loneliness Wenger and Burholt (2004) develop a typology to classify the changing patterns of isolation demonstrated by their group. They report that 43 per cent had a stable pattern of isolation at each follow-up point: 26 per cent were never classified as isolated whilst 17 per cent were isolated at each time point. Only a minority, two per cent, overcame isolation, 15 per cent fluctuated and 28 per cent became isolated. For 13 per cent the index could not be computed because of missing data. Clearly further studies are needed to determine how representative these patterns are to the general population. However, they do indicate that, as with loneliness, single-point-in-time studies do not fully represent the dynamic nature of the experience and that patterns of loneliness and isolation are not fixed but are subject to change in response to changing circumstances and the social situation within which older people find themselves.

As we have suggested several times the varying ways that isolation indices have been measured does pose problems for comparative analyses. As with our focus upon loneliness we are interested in how the extent of isolation may (or may not) have changed over time. Table 5.3 does provide this information but the variability of measures means that we can only draw preliminary and tentative conclusions. We would argue that this table demonstrates that most older people are not isolated – regardless of measure used – and that if we focus upon the 'severe' group this seems to be fairly stable over time at 5–15 per cent. However, further conclusions and inferences cannot be drawn from this table as it would be too speculative. A key question for our project was how have levels of isolation changed in the past 50 years? The data presented in this chapter suggest a pattern of stability rather than one of rapid increase. The percentage of older people who are severely isolated ranges from 10–15 per cent whilst the percentage defined as 'not isolated' – with the exception of the study by Scharf – is around 60–70 per cent. Hence the majority of older people are not isolated – this is a minority experience just as was the case with loneliness and again the pattern is one of broad stability over time. There seems to be little evidence to support a 'moral panic' concerning the social disengagement of older people.

## Conclusion: the link between loneliness and isolation

Thus far we have focused upon loneliness and isolation as separate concepts. In addition, we have sought to locate these 'pathological' dimensions of social engagement in later life within a broad context of a focus upon the overall patterns of social participation and engagement demonstrated by older people to reinforce the message that most older people are socially engaged in a variety of different ways. We have demonstrated that both loneliness and isolation are a minority experience and that they illustrate differing trajectories across the life course. Although, as we argued in Chapter 1, loneliness and isolation are two distinct concepts the terms are often used interchangeably. In this final section we consider the degree of inter-relationship between these two 'pathological' dimensions of social engagement. The conceptual distinction between isolation and loneliness was noted by Townsend (1957) in his survey of east London where he proposed a four-fold typology:

* lonely but not isolated

* isolated but not lonely

* lonely and isolated

* neither.

This typology was subsequently developed and used by Tunstall (1966) and more recently by Wenger and Burholt (2004). Whilst this is conceptually clear, operationalising this typology is problematic because of decisions as to how the 'intermediate' categories of loneliness and isolation are attributed and by how we measure the two concepts. Should the intermediate categories of 'sometimes' lonely be included as 'lonely' or 'not lonely'? Similarly, are those classified as illustrating modest levels of isolation to be classified as isolated or not isolated? These are important decisions because they will obviously influence the size and composition of the groups and may lead to erroneous conclusions being drawn about them and, potentially, inappropriate interventions being developed.

For our study we had four categories of loneliness and four categories of isolation. As we have seen previously in this and the preceding chapter there are few people in the most severe grouping for each variable – two per cent respectively being classed as severely lonely/ isolated. Hence the two top categories were grouped together to define the severe lonely/isolated category. We retain this grouping throughout this analysis. Given the ambiguity of the 'sometimes' category for loneliness and the definition of the 'lowest' category of isolation on the basis of a single response we have undertaken the analysis using two different approaches. In the first we have allocated these two groups to the 'not lonely/not isolated' categories respectively. Using this approach the majority of our participants, 69 per cent, were defined as neither lonely nor isolated, 22 per cent were isolated, six per cent were lonely and three per cent were both lonely and isolated (see Table 5.5).

We accept, however, that the typology is very sensitive to the allocative decisions made and it is worth demonstrating how this

**Table 5.5** The relationship between loneliness and isolation

| Study | Lonely & isolated | Lonely | Isolated | None |
|---|---|---|---|---|
| Townsend[1] | 1 | 4 | 9 | 86 |
| Tunstall[2] | 5 | 6 | 22 | 69 |
| ESRC Survey | 3 | 6 | 22 | 69 |
| ESRC Survey | 35 | 12 | 42 | 11 |

*Sources:* 1. Townsend (1957)
       2. Tunstall (1966)

influences the results. By allocating the lowest category of loneliness/ isolation into the 'case' category we alter the distribution massively. This would give us only 11 per cent of our population as neither isolated nor lonely; 35 per cent both isolated and lonely; 12 per cent as lonely and 42 per cent as isolated (see Table 5.5). This suggests that the definitions are being drawn much too tightly – the 'normal' experience is being pathologised and defined as abnormal or deviant in terms of being either isolated or lonely. This is somewhat parallel to including living alone as a measure of loneliness or isolation – it is too insensitive because the characteristic is shared by too many of the study population. Hence for the subsequent analyses we allocated our intermediate categories to the non-isolated/lonely categories.

We applied our scoring algorithm of allocating the intermediate categories to the not lonely/isolated because of the ambiguity of their derivation from the data presented by previous studies. This reveals that the vast majority of older people, 88 per cent in Townsend's study, 76 per cent in Tunstall's study and 69 per cent in the ESRC survey are defined as neither lonely nor isolated. Furthermore, the percentage classed as both has remained consistently small over the five decades separating the fieldwork for these studies and the relationship between the categories is largely unchanged (see Table 5.5). The separation of our population into distinct categories supports the assertion that, overall, loneliness and isolation are predominantly separate and distinct categories with only limited overlap between them. The identification of two distinct sets of 'risk factors' for these two experiences further supports the argument that they are distinct social entities with separate causal pathways, which would require differing remedial interventions.

In this chapter we have looked at social isolation conceptualised in various guises as a broad measure of social engagement, total social contacts or as a composite index based upon availability of and contact with family and friends. This has been located within a broad framework of social exclusion as defined by Scharf and Smith (2004). We can draw several conclusions from our analysis. First, it is noticeable from the interview data that older people conceptualised isolation in terms of social or spatial distance from their local communities. Some commented upon ideas of geographical isolation – being distant from towns or places where activities and people were located. Others commented upon how the impact of neighbourhood change had served to isolate them. These comments remind us of the importance of the sense of place and the physical importance of space and location in facilitating older people to remain socially engaged and active members of family and community groups.

We argued at the beginning of this book that loneliness and isolation are two distinct and discrete social entities. This position is supported by two aspects of our analyses. First, if we examine the overlap between these social phenomena then there are only a small minority who demonstrate both isolation and loneliness. This is a feature that we can also observe in the work of Tunstall and Townsend. Second, when we examine the factors that predispose older people to loneliness and isolation, then there is only limited overlap between them. Loneliness is predicted by time alone and perceptions of health and old age. Isolation is associated with the availability of a social network, the availability of help and presence of a confidante and social emeddedness as indicated by knowing and trusting neighbours. This links back to our participants' comments about the sense that isolation is social detachment from the locality in which they live. This suggests that developing community links could be one way of helping alleviate isolation across the age groups. Given the difficulties of defining and identifying the 'isolated' then perhaps the most effective way of combating this is to target community development more generally and this will benefit members across the generations.

# 6

# Rethinking loneliness and social isolation in later life

There are many myths and stereotypes surrounding the experience of ageing and later life. For example, we readily conceptualise old age as a time of universal and inevitable biological decline that then manifests itself in physical and mental frailty (Victor, 2005; Mulley, 2007). Additionally we also perceive older people as being neglected and marginalised by society; in more current policy parlance, we see them as 'socially excluded'. Combined with a negative perception of the contemporary experience of old age we also hark back to a time when older people were cherished and valued and were firmly integrated with the social fabric of their communities. We see loneliness and isolation as largely associated with later life. For example, an article by Killen (1998) published in the *Journal of Advanced Nursing* was entitled 'Loneliness: an epidemic in modern society'. Whilst not specifically about older people it encapsulates, if unintentionally, the way that we think about the extent to which older people experience this phenomenon. As Sheldon wrote 'Loneliness is a well known calamity of old age' (1948 p. 127). In the research that underpins this volume we sought to examine some of the redolent stereotypes that focus on the social exclusion of older people and the perception that things are much 'worse' than they used to be. We wanted to: (a) look at the relationship between different concepts such as loneliness and isolation, (b) look at trends in terms of the extent to which such experiences where becoming more (or less) common within contemporary British society and (c) look at how these experiences within Britain compared with other countries. In this final chapter we consider the answers to these three questions and consider some of the policy, practice and research responses to our findings.

## Terminological inexactitute – distinguishing the key concepts

It is not uncommon to see and hear the terms 'loneliness' and 'isolation' used interchangeably. Furthermore, other related terms like 'living alone' or 'being alone' are also used to mean loneliness and isolation rather than being descriptions of living arrangements or time spent alone respectively. However, the academic literature draws a clear theoretical, conceptual and operational distinction between these states. Loneliness and isolation are two related but distinct experiences, which have distinct associated factors, require distinct policy responses and which may well have distinct causal pathways. A key dimension of our research has been to differentiate these concepts and determine the degree of overlap between them. In this section we look at each of four key concepts (loneliness, social isolation, living alone and being alone) individually and examine the degree of overlap and thereby determine if, indeed, we can use one as a proxy for another.

### Loneliness

Loneliness is an essentially subjective experience and, perhaps, one that we all experience. It is part of the experience of being human. As Rokach (1990: 39) states 'loneliness is as natural and integral a part of being human as are joy, hunger and self actualisation' further stating that 'humans are born alone, they experience the terror of loneliness in death and often much loneliness in between'. Whilst we do not accept his entire proposition, especially the presumption around death and dying, this is a useful exposition on the essential universal nature of loneliness. Central to our work have been the ideas that loneliness is not exclusive to older people and that it is not exclusive to Britain.

Our starting point has been that loneliness is a subjective experience. As such this poses, for the empirical social scientist, problems of how such an essentially personal experience can de defined and then measured. We consider loneliness to be the gap between the desired or expected level of social interaction and the actual level. Hence this is a relativist construct that is unique to each individual and their situation. As such it may vary between people, for the same person at different points in their lives and both within and between societies. This therefore makes cohort, age-related and inter-country comparisons problematic.

Our approach to measuring loneliness was influenced by our definitional stance (and our desire to make historical comparisons). Consequently we have used a 'single-question self-rating' scale that requires individuals to evaluate their current level of loneliness. Clearly this requires individuals, in an interview situation, to report the existence of a highly negatively evaluated state of mind to an interviewer. Analysis of our survey data and those from related studies suggest that older people (and probably others) are perfectly able and willing to answer such questions. In Chapter 2, however, we highlighted how survey participants may express the 'public account' (Cornwell, 1984) of later life and conform to the perceived expectations of survey interviewers rather than 'private accounts' and perhaps accounts that more honestly reflect their personal lives. In our interview survey only two participants declined to answer this and other studies have reported similarly good rates of response. In very broad terms, the single self-rating style question to assess loneliness seems broadly acceptable. We may contrast this with some of the longer scales where the overall rating may be compromised by missing data. For example, using the de Jong scale in a postal survey in Perth resulted in 53 out of 352 participants (15 per cent) being excluded from the analysis. Furthermore, we know that this pattern of item omission is not random. In the Perth study the non-response bias was toward women and people in the older age groups (see Victor et al., 2005a). We may speculate that other studies that use composite scales to measure loneliness may experience similar problems with item omission thereby potentially increasing non-response bias and limiting the generalisability of the findings.

Leaving aside the issue of respondent acceptability as defined by item omission, does it matter which type of measure is used to establish the extent of loneliness in later life? There are few studies that have directly investigated this issue and most of these have focused on comparing the properties of differing versions of the same instrument and there is much more interest in this issue in the literature investigating loneliness in childhood (Goossens and Beyers, 2002). The study by Victor and colleagues (Victor et al., 2005a) is one of the few that has examined the utility of differing measures of loneliness with an older population and which has directly compared self-report and composite measures. On the basis of this study we suggest that in terms of identifying the 'severely' lonely and the definitely 'not lonely' groups (i.e. the two extremes of the distribution) then there is probably little variation between measures (Victor et al., 2005a). Where the self-report and composite scales diverge is in the intermediate categories. This probably reflects the intersection of two factors. First, for the self-report measures the category 'sometimes' is problematic and would probably benefit from greater definitional clarity (although none of our respondents found this problematic); it is likely that a category such as 'sometimes' could be subject to slippage in meaning over time. Second, for the composite scales the size of the intermediate categories of loneliness is greatly influenced by where the boundaries are drawn along the continuum of scores. However, this is clearly an area where there is considerable potential for further work.

A key objective for us was to investigate what, if any, changes there were in the experience of loneliness across differing cohorts of older people. As we have demonstrated (see Victor et al., 2002) there appears to be little strong or compelling evidence to suggest that we are either experiencing an epidemic of loneliness in old age or that rates of loneliness have increased markedly over time. Self-reported significant loneliness ('very/often lonely') is experienced by about 5–15 per cent of the population aged 65 years and over and this has remained stable over the past 60 years (Wenger et al., 1996). Over the same period studies have demonstrated an association between clinical depression and loneliness (Wenger et al., 1996). Contemporary data, however, suggest that this is not synonymous with depression or acting as a proxy for sub-clinical or borderline depression. Using our main comparator studies summarised in Chapter 4 we can observe a decrease in the percentage of people describing themselves as 'not lonely' from about three-quarters to two-thirds over 50 years (see Table 4.2). So, despite this decrease, which might reflect a 'real' change or the imprecision of the intermediate 'sometimes lonely' category, the majority of people at any specific point in time are not lonely.

Across northern European countries, North America and Australasia rates of loneliness are broadly comparable with the levels described in our study and reviewed in detail in Chapter 4. Given the changing family structures characteristic of these countries it is, perhaps, not surprising to see this interest in researching loneliness. Perhaps more surprising is the emergence of research examining loneliness in later life from Latin American and Asian countries (Joia et al., 2007; Chen et al., 2004), where we might presume such concerns are less prominent. In particular, the 'one-child policy' and rapid economic change experienced in China has disproportionately affected older people. This has stimulated academic research such as the study examining loneliness amongst Chinese elders by Zhang and Liu (2007). Respondents were asked if they were 'lonely and isolated' – never, seldom, sometimes and often/always. Eight per cent of Chinese elders reported that they were always lonely and isolated – a similar proportion to our study – while 24 per cent were in the 'sometimes' category. Such reports have prompted comments such as the following: 'What the old people need, more than money, is more emotional support from their children' (Peng Zhenqiu, NPC deputy from Shanghai). 'More calls and visits are necessary to resolve old people's loneliness' (*China Daily*, 2006). The wide range of studies about loneliness indicate that whilst culturally mediated, it is an experience that is universally identifiable amongst populations of older people and, presumably, younger people as well.

We have also demonstrated the complexity of the differing categories included within prevalence-based studies of loneliness. Single time-point studies identify a group of people as lonely (or isolated) but do not usually deconstruct this category into component parts. In our qualitative interviews we were able to distinguish three broad groups within the category of lonely: those for whom it was a new (or worsening) experience; those for whom it was decreasing; and those for whom it was an enduring feature of life. Whilst our study was not a longitudinal design we were able to reconstruct these categories by asking participants to consider their perceptions of social relations 10 years before. The results were broadly similar with the few longitudinal studies that have been published. Clearly the precise details are contingent upon the measure used to identify loneliness but broadly 50–60 per cent of those aged 65 or over were not lonely and had not experienced loneliness; 12–15 per cent had experienced this persistently over the life course; 5–10 per cent reported less loneliness with age and the remaining 20–25 per cent reported that it gets worse. Studies with multiple follow-up points such as those by Wenger and Burholt (2004) identify a 'fluctuating' group as well. We would argue that the persistently lonely group are intrinsically different from the other two groups of people who report loneliness. The latter seems to be a reaction to changes in the individuals' life courses such as widowhood or changing social norms where a broadly ageist, youth orientated society can make older people 'seem invisible' (Sinclair et al., 2007). If we accept this distinction then this has considerable implications for the development of policies designed to ameliorate loneliness specifically and exclusion more broadly. We examine these issues later in this chapter.

## Isolation

In Chapter 2 we examined the complexity inherent in the notion of social isolation. We can distinguish from the literature a variety of differing conceptualisations including: the deprivation of intimacy and companionship; absence or low levels of social contact; lack of social networks or support; social inadequacy; feelings of 'otherness'; feelings of isolation and loneliness. Hence within the broad term of isolation we have two distinct manifestations including an 'empirical' aspect relating to ideas about number of contacts, size of social networks and the ability to translate these into active social support and an individual's feelings about themselves in terms of their social adequacy (or rather perceived inadequacies or detachment). In our study we have adopted the more empirical approach by examining total contacts and aspects of the social network within which the individual is embedded. This enables us to both adopt an historical approach and develop our 'cohort comparison' to examine the continuities and changes within the experience of ageing.

However, there is another dimension to isolation that researchers have not traditionally incorporated but which was prominent in our interviews and is also a theme evident in a recent Help the Aged publication on social inclusion (Owen, 2007; Sinclair et al., 2007). Both these publications and our interviewees stressed the important of geographical isolation but the notion of the spatial element of isolation has been very largely excluded from the body of work concerned with isolation in later life. There is some research examining the feelings of isolation that result from the geographical separateness of the places in which older people live, especially those living in care homes. Sinclair et al. (2007) draw attention to the 'separateness' of care homes and that this can produce feelings of being 'cut off or remote' from society; as if such residences are no longer part of the mainstream of society. Geographical isolation is, however, also experienced at the individual level. For example, one of Sinclair et al.'s participants commented 'I still feel part of society but the lack of mobility hinders this' (Sinclair et al., 2007: 32) whilst another commented, 'you can't get out, you can't go anywhere' (Sinclair et al., 2007: 33). The spatial dimension of isolation may also be reinforced by other factors which result in the boundaries of an older person's environment becoming more constrained, such as fear of crime, infrequent transport, poor street lighting plus environmental factors both man-made such as busy roads or natural such as hills. As one of our participants commented in response to the question 'Do you ever feel isolated?':

> Isolated? Mmmmmm no, we have a bus now if we need to give out anywhere. I have a bus stop right outside here you see so I'm lucky. [209: 5: 37–9]

Place is clearly important for the experience of later life and, indeed, for other age groups as well. There is much scope to develop and integrate the social and spatial elements of isolation when examining the social world of older people (Peace et al., 2006).

We can identify another element to the feelings of isolation that has consistently emerged in both our study and recent community studies (Sinclair et al., 2007; Phillipson et al., 2001) and that is the sense that neighbourhoods and communities have changed around them leaving the older people as isolated survivors of a previous generation. Almost inevitably such changes in the composition of the local community, whether based upon changes in the age or ethnic structure of the locality, are viewed negatively. Such changes can threaten or compromise the place attachment of older people by threatening their feelings of 'togetherness' with their locality, their recognition and familiarity and their sense of control (Peace et al., 2006). It is not just change in the socio-demographic fabric of neighbours that is contributing to feelings of social isolation but also the pace of social change and innovation. Two participants in Sinclair et al.'s study summed up these issues neatly with their comments: 'Lots of things happen today that I don't know about or understand and I feel cut off' and 'I think that life is getting very fast for older people and it's getting worse – it's all very complicated'. Or as one of our participants reported:

I think of age as a sort of cultural phenomenon, things seem strange. Like a lot of television advertising. I think I don't understand that now, that must be because there's something I'm supposed to see that I've missed, I don't understand. [203: 9: 47–9]

Whilst there is evidence that older people are engaging more actively with the consumption and lifestyle-based elements of contemporary society, this is not a universal experience (Higgs and Gilleard, 2006) and there is a 'digital divide' emerging between those with access to the on-line world and those without.

Hence our empirical survey material uses a fairly conventional approach to the measurement of isolation, defined both in terms of the existence of a social network and the quantification of a contact score. We accept that this approach is limited. It neither takes account of the quality aspect of the relationships implied by the existence of contacts and family, nor does it include either the important spatial component or the qualitative external factors of neighbourhood and social change. We would thus argue that there is considerable scope in conceptual, methodological and empirical arenas for developing our understanding of isolation in later life.

## Living alone

Perhaps one of the most fundamental changes in the experience of later life in Britain since 1945 has been the increase in older people living alone. Prior to 1945 there were few older people who lived either alone or just with their spouse. The majority lived in extended, two-plus generation households. This is no longer the case with most people aged 65 years or over living either alone or with their spouse. To put this into context in the 1800 survey of York only 10 per cent of those aged 60 years or over lived alone. Nowadays younger people increasingly set up their own home before marriage or establishing a long-term relationship. In 1971, 18 per cent of all households in Great Britain consisted of a single person; by 2006 this had risen to 29 per cent comprising some 7 million people. In addition to the numerical and proportional increase the nature of people living in these types of households has changed. In 1971 two-thirds of single-person households were classified as pensioners, whilst by 2005 this had reduced to 50 per cent (Fido et al., 2006). Hence half of all single-person households are now made up of people under the age of retirement. Consequently, the household category 'living alone' covers a much wider spectrum of the population than it did even three decades ago. For current generations of older people their only experience of living alone may well come about when they are widowed in later life. Future generations may well have experienced a period of living alone much earlier in their life course which may (or may not) change the nature of the experience of living alone in later life.

Living and being alone is, however, easily problematised. Part of the attraction of using living alone as a symbolic representation of a variety of social ills such as isolation, exclusion, poverty, neglect and abuse is that it is a readily available measure. Furthermore, as the measure is available for a long(ish) historical time span it is comparatively easy to demonstrate the increase in living alone and, by extension, isolation, exclusion and loneliness. The simple linkage between living alone and loneliness and neglect is illustrated by the 'one is the saddest number' campaign run by Help the Aged for Christmas 2006 (http://www.saddestnumber.org.uk/). Whilst we have no wish to denigrate the good work done by Help the Aged, such campaigns can help to perpetuate the presumption that living alone is in itself a problem and that there is a direct link with loneliness and isolation. This is illustrated by the headline 'Britain singled out as a lonely nation because there are more single-person households and fewer marriages' (http://news.-bbc.co.uk/1/hi/uk/692150.stm). However, the stereotype does not just apply to Britain as this comment on the latest US census indicates: 'For all its crowds, Manhattan may also be the country's loneliest metropolis. It has the highest percentage of single-person households of any county in the nation, according to the US Census Bureau' (http://www.usatoday.com/news/nation/2005-09-02-living-alone_x.htm). Again, the presumption is made that living lone equates to loneliness, isolation and exclusion.

As our project has comprehensively demonstrated, there is no statistically significant link between living alone and loneliness and isolation when other related factors are taken into account. It is true that loneliness and isolation are more common amongst those who live alone than those who live in larger family groups or households. This was noted by Sheldon (1948) and Townsend (1957). However, once we take into account the other attributes of those living alone, such as widowhood, then it is evident that it is these factors that are important in the development of loneliness and not living alone per se. This is emphasised in the work looking at changes in loneliness over time. As Thompson (1973 p. 887) wrote 'Living alone need not mean isolation – it is often possible to feel more isolated in the midst of a family.' Yet despite such statements and research revealing the complexity of the relationship between living alone, loneliness and isolation, the presumption of a link between living arrangements and social relationships persists. Indeed this presumption is demonstrated by the inclusion of 'living alone' as a component factor in many measures of social isolation. As we demonstrated in Chapter 5, the inclusion of this measures results in very high levels of isolation and the 'pathologising' of virtually all the population aged 65 years and over.

## How has the experience of living alone changed for older people?

Loneliness, isolation and loneliness are all more common amongst those who live alone. Our data indicate that, of those living alone, 17 per cent reported that they were often or always lonely compared with two per cent living in larger household groups. Looked at another way, 87 per cent of those who were often or always lonely lived alone (see Table 6.1). Superficially this looks like very strong evidence to support the presumed link between loneliness and living alone. Such relationships are, however, associations and we must not rush to imply (explicitly or implicitly) a causal link. As we noted in our analysis living alone is itself associated with other demographic factors that are linked with loneliness and isolation such as advanced age, widowhood and being female. Once we take these factors into account living alone ceases to become an important predictive factor. Whilst it is easy to see how a link may be made between living alone and loneliness and isolation we must resist this temptation and look at the factors underlying this link. As noted above it is predominantly widowhood that is linked with loneliness and not living alone per se. Hence it is the disruption of an established way of life and social links that is a key factor.

Whilst we strongly argue that living alone is not of itself a risk factor for loneliness other researchers have arrived at different conclusions. Whilst there is almost universal consensus of an established relationship in studies restricted to univariate analysis, the situation is less clear cut for studies using multivariate analyses. As we reported in Chapter 4 our results are unusual in that seven out of the eight studies reviewed identified living alone as an independent risk factor. However, as our review indicates there is considerable variation in the type of modelling used to undertake these analyses and in the variables included in the models. Hence it is hardly surprising that there is variation across studies in the risk factors identified. More specifically our study was unusual in including a measure of time spent alone and, potentially, the living alone measure used by other researchers could have been acting as a proxy for this.

From a health promotion or public health policy perspective the commonly assumed link between loneliness or isolation with living alone is very useful. In developing screening tools to identify those 'at risk' of experiencing these negative states then living alone is an easy measure to define and identify. It is comparatively easy to assess and categorise household size and, as such, this variable is very attractive as a mechanism for identifying 'at risk' elders. Living alone has been associated with a variety of negative health and quality of life variables in both Britain (Kharicha et al., 2007) and elsewhere (Yeh and Lo, 2004a). In terms of sensitivity and specificity, criteria used in public health to assess the utility of disease-based screening measures, living alone is a poor variable. Because living alone in later life is so common, inclusion of living alone as part of a (or the only) screening tool would result in large numbers of 'false positives'. That is people who live alone and are not isolated or lonely but are identified by the tool as being at risk. The tool cannot precisely identify those who are lonely and therefore has low sensitivity.

However, a variety of researchers are 'looking behind' the single category of living alone to consider the complexity of this social category (Ogg, 2003; Luken and Vaughan, 2003) and the web of relationships within which those living alone may be enmeshed. For example, a recent study by Walker and Hiller (2007) has demonstrated that older women who live alone can have extensive social and support networks that they use to develop and maintain their independence. Again, in this study there is an important contextualising and enabling (or disabling) role played by the nature and characteristics of the local neighbourhood.

Living alone is not necessarily evaluated negatively by our older participants, as this interview extract illustrates:

> Q: And do you like living alone?
>
> A: I don't, you say do I like living alone ... obviously I'd rather my husband were alive. Apart from that yes I do, I think I'd prefer to live alone rather than to live with anybody else. [303: 2: 20–4]

Whilst for those who have been widowed it is clearly not a positive choice it is, perhaps, a living arrangement that is preferable to any other alternatives, as this extract illustrates:

> Q: Do you like living alone?
>
> A: Well let me say, at my age I'd rather be here than in a home. That's the alternative. What is the alternative? Living alone, or going into sheltered accommodation I mean there's not much.
>
> Q: Would you consider living with one of your children?
>
> A: Oh no, not that, oh no, you can't land yourself on them, that would be the end of a relationship straightaway I should think. Unless there was a lot of land and you could build a little bungalow or something. Something entirely separate, but it couldn't be in the same building. You could go into a flat in somebody else's house but I don't think that would work.
>
> Q: So you live alone now through circumstance rather than through choice?
>
> A: Oh yes. [202: 7: 4–20]

By targeting interventions at this group service providers are treating those living alone as a single homogeneous group. This is far from the case. Within the category of older people living alone are people who are recently widowed, the 'established' widowed, those who have always lived alone plus all the other attributes that differentiate populations such as gender, class, ethnicity, health, age and status. In particular, we contrast the experience of those for whom living alone is a 'new' experience and those for whom it is an established way of life or one that they may have experienced earlier in the life course. For women in their 80s widowhood may well herald major changes in household circumstances and one that they may never previously have experienced. For many women (or men) in this age group they would have lived with either parents (or in-laws) after marriage before establishing their own independent household. It is unlikely that men and women in this age group ever 'lived alone'. We can contrast this with both older people who have always lived alone and younger cohorts for whom living alone may well have been part of their early adulthood experiences. All of these factors will intersect to shape an individual's experience of living alone in later life and their predisposition (or otherwise) to loneliness and isolation. To treat all of these people as at risk of either loneliness or isolation is naïve and policy solutions based upon using living arrangements or household size as a proxy for social exclusion are unlikely to succeed.

## Being alone

'Now I'm all alone and that's the only way to be' is a line from 'Meet on the ledge' written by Richard Thompson. Being alone is, as we suggested earlier, presumed to be both a predisposing factor for loneliness and isolation and virtually co-terminus with living alone. As with living alone, the concept of 'being alone' is a straightforward characterisation of how much time individuals spend by themselves. In our survey 47 per cent of participants reported that they were always or often alone with 10 per cent indicating that they were never alone.

In their research both Townsend (1957) and Tunstall (1966) linked the time individuals spent alone with loneliness and isolation. Again, our survey reproduced these associations when we looked at time spent alone in relation to both self-report levels of loneliness and our three measures of isolation. Of those who reported that they were often or always alone, 18 per cent were always or often lonely. Looked at the other way, 90 per cent of those who were often or always lonely reported that they were always or often alone. In our multivariate analyses when we controlled for confounding factors such as widowhood we found that the relationship was maintained. Spending large amounts of time alone is, for the general population of older people, an independent risk factor for loneliness. Ours is the only study that has identified this relationship when using a multivariate statistical model to interrogate the data. We are not clear if this is because other studies have not included this variable or if the relationship is not statistically robust. We feel that exploring the role of time spent alone with regard to loneliness and isolation might be more fruitful than the more commonly preferred living alone variable. However, time spent alone did not translate into a link with isolation. In order to understand this relationship we can examine the characteristics of those who spend significant amounts of time alone.

Like loneliness and isolation the amount of time spent alone by older people is not equally distributed within the population. Women, those living alone, the 'not married' and the older members of the population are the groups who reported higher than average rates of time spent alone. For example, 12 per cent of those participants classified as married reported that they were often or always alone compared with 70 per cent or over for those in all other marital status categories. Similarly, those who live alone, not surprisingly, reported high rates of being alone (80 per cent for those living alone compared with 14 per cent for those living with others). There is a relationship with both age and gender but this is less marked and largely reflects variability in the 'often' category of time spent alone. Four per cent of both men and women reported that they were always alone, but 38 per cent of women reported that they were often alone compared with 28 per cent of men. No significant relationships were observed with our measures of social and material resources and there was a very weak link to physical health. Unlike loneliness and isolation, but more like living alone, the main links between time spent alone are with the socio-demographic factors, most notably marital status and household size; there was little obvious relationships with our other factors. Hence time spent alone is of limited utility as a measure of social engagement but it obviously links to loneliness and isolation via the very strong relationships with marital status and household size.

We had only a limited opportunity to explore the issue of aloneness as distinct from being or living alone. However, we think that the concept of aloneness in later life is an under-researched area. Whilst we have established quantitative estimates of the broad categories of time older people spend alone we have not fully explored notions of aloneness. Pierce et al. (2003) report, in their study of older women being treated for depression, how the meaning of aloneness can vary as their participants recovered from depression. Initially aloneness was seen in a highly negative way being characterised as representing vulnerability, helplessness and loss of identity. As their depression lifted aloneness was seen as representing self-reliance, resourcefulness and self-determination; a set of highly positive characteristics. Clearly aloneness has not been researched as much as some of the other topic areas we have dealt with in this book. However, we think it is an important topic for further research, especially as it is so clearly linked with the day-to-day experience of later life. It is also important because of the obvious variability in meaning that can be attached to it. It is not hard to imagine health and social care professionals construing the aloneness of an older person in a highly negative fashion and to see it as a manifestation of vulnerability and a reason to intervene in the life of that person. In contrast the older person might, like the participants in Pierce et al.'s (2003) study, see it as a manifestation of their independence and autonomy. Hence it is important that in such professionally based encounters both groups establish that they are attributing a common meaning to such concepts as aloneness, isolation and loneliness.

## Loneliness, isolation, living alone and being alone: separate states or co-terminus concepts?

In summary, therefore, what is the degree of overlap between these four dimensions? As Table 6.1 illustrates, the largest percentage of those classified as often or sometimes lonely are those who are living alone (87 per cent) or spend a significant amount of their time alone (90 per cent). This is much higher than the percentages derived from earlier studies, although given the great increase in the percentage of

**Table 6.1** The inter-relationship between loneliness, living alone, being alone and isolation

|  | % who are often/always lonely | % of the often/always lonely | % of the often/always lonely Tunstall[1] | % of the often/always lonely Sheldon[2] |
|---|---|---|---|---|
| Living alone | 14 | 87 | 53 | 41 |
| Often/ always alone | 16 | 90 | ** | ** |
| Isolated | 12 | 46 | ** | ** |

*Notes:* **Not available
*Sources:* 1. Sheldon (1948), 2. Tunstall (1966)

people living alone (which has tripled since the studies of Tunstall and Sheldon) is not unexpected. However, as this table indicates, whilst living alone and being alone are greatly over-represented in the category defined as lonely this still remains a minority experience amongst those living alone or those who spend a substantial amount of time alone.

## Predicting loneliness and isolation

As well as exploring the specific links between loneliness and isolation and living and being alone we wished to examine the relationship between these two states and a broader range of factors. We classified individual variables into four broad groupings: socio-demographic; health resources; social resources and material resources. Here we focus upon the key robust relationships that emerged from our analysis of the data using multivariate analysis.

### Socio-demographic factors

In the earlier sections we have noted on several occasions the important link between loneliness and widowhood when discussing the complexity of the variable 'living alone'. This has been comprehensively established in our study with 20 per cent of widows or widowers classifying themselves as always or often lonely. Some 85 per cent of those who were often or always lonely were widowed. This relationship was maintained in the multivariate analysis and is reported by seven out of the eight studies reviewed. Similarly, widowhood was linked with isolation as measured in terms of both total social contacts and the Scharf index. The observed relationship between widowhood and both isolation and loneliness therefore seems robust. Indeed this is reinforced by the available longitudinal studies of loneliness where widowhood emerges as key factor. This was also recognised by our participants where the primacy of the marital relationship and the consequences for loneliness were often commented on. For example:

> B: But the only thing is we don't get lonely because we've got each other. (they hold hands) If we were alone, either one of us, I think we would be very lonely because there would be no...
>
> A: Almost suicidal I would guess. [103: 6: 30–4]

Most studies indicate that there is an initial link between loneliness and gender (see Beal, 2006, for an overview). Whilst reported levels of loneliness were higher amongst women than men in our study, 11 per cent versus eight per cent, this was not maintained when our multivariate analysis was done. As Victor et al. (2005c) report, loneliness is not an exclusively female affair with a ratio of approximately 60:40 in terms of absolute numbers. Scaling this up to the general population of elders suggests that there are a considerable number of lonely men in the population and that both policy and practice need to recognise this diversity. Indeed, examination of the studies using multivariate analyses indicates that only one out the eight studies identified an independent link between loneliness and gender whilst there was no link evident with isolation.

In a similar vein our findings regarding the link between age and loneliness are, perhaps on first sight, somewhat controversial. Our preliminary analysis indicates that the reported extent of loneliness increases from six per cent at age 65–74 to 18 per cent at age 85 years and over. However, because of the small number of individuals interviewed in the older age group only 13 per cent of all those reporting themselves as lonely were aged 85 years and over. Once the influence of other variables was taken into account the multivariate analysis produced a rather intriguing finding that suggested advanced age was 'protective' against loneliness and that some older people were 'overcoming loneliness'. To the best of our knowledge this finding is both unique to our study and very intriguing. It suggests that with increasing age there is the potential for positive change. This is a contrast to the rather prevalent bio-medical paradigm of universal and inevitable age-related decline.

## Material resources

The predictive model that we used enabled us to identify not just 'risk or vulnerability' factors but also 'protective' factors. We have already noted the potentially ameliorating effects of advanced age indicative of an adaptive mechanism. Our analysis also identified that several proxy variables for material resources (home ownership, access to a car and possession of educational qualifications) were associated with lower levels of loneliness. One of these, educational qualifications, was statistically significant albeit only just making the five per cent level. So whilst we would not wish to overstate this relationship because of the marginality of the relation several other studies have linked levels of loneliness with measures (and proxy measures) of material resources. This is clearly an area that merits further research and some support for the importance of this topic is the relationship between low income and loneliness identified by Savikko et al. (2005). There are far fewer studies that have used a multivariate statistical approach to the study of isolation. Hence we have fewer studies with which to compare our results and findings of a link between car ownership and isolation. Wenger (1996) has noted a relationship between isolation and class which is supportive of our findings. However, for our participants finances were very important for maintaining social engagement and thereby combating loneliness and isolation, as this interview extract illustrates:

> A: I should think another thing is if one's financial circumstances are not very good this must have a bearing on what you can do. Living on the basic pension I think one could find that you're out, your contact with other people is not very good, because the basic state pension is very low indeed.
>
> B: You'd spend all your money on just surviving.
>
> A: It does make a difference. And going to see family, if your family lives ... when our son was here he and his wife lived the other side of Cheltenham. Now that's two bus journeys from here. You have to go in to Cheltenham and out the other side where they live and that was expensive. I mean I used to do it on my bike. But if you had to take two buses how often would you be able to do that? [203: 6: 27–41]

## Health resources

We examined the relationship between loneliness, isolation and a variety of health variables. Initially we reported links between loneliness and seven health factors including limiting long-standing illness, disability, problems with sight/hearing, health rating, health expectations of old age and mental ill-health (the GHQ 12). Such relationships have been reported by previous studies and there is a substantial body of work linking loneliness with a variety of bio-medical markers and negative health outcomes including dementia (Wilson et al., 2007).

Previous research has focused on the relationship between loneliness and depression. The GHQ used in our study is not a measure of depression; rather it focuses upon general psychiatric morbidity. However, it demonstrates the same relationship with loneliness as depression does. Rates of loneliness were 25 per cent for those with severe psychiatric morbidity levels and eight per cent for those with a moderate level of psychiatric morbidity as 'measured' by the GHQ. Of those who are lonely, 57 per cent had severe or moderate morbidity. Although there exists an association between psychiatric morbidity and loneliness, psychiatric morbidity (particularly depression) and loneliness should be treated as distinct phenomena and not reported as the same. Of those categorised as having severe psychiatric morbidity using the GHQ (255 participants) 60 per cent had an elevated psychiatric morbidity only, 16 per cent were lonely but were not categorised as having severe psychiatric morbidity and 21 per cent were both. Hence the overlap, whilst important, is only for a minority of participants.

None of the physical health-related factors retained their importance in the multivariate analysis. Few other studies report an association between physical health and loneliness. This may be because they did not include the spectrum of variables that characterise physical and mental well-being. However, it is noteworthy that five out of eight studies reported a positive association between disability, chronic health or poor functional ability and loneliness. Three health-related variables were included in our final model for the 'prediction' of loneliness: psychiatric morbidity, self-rated subjective health and expectations of health in old age. Self-rated health demonstrates an independent association with loneliness in every study reviewed except that reported by Jylhä (2004). In our study 19 per cent of those who rated their health as poor reported that they were often or always lonely. Our study also included a variable relating to how people's health in 'old age' had lived up to their expectations. Overall 27 per cent of our participants reported that their health was worse than they had expected and 30 per cent that it was better. Those who rated their health worse than expected reported significantly higher rates of loneliness than those who rated it better (15 per cent versus 8 per cent) and this association was maintained in the multivariate analysis. In addition, deterioration in health rating has been linked with loneliness in longitudinal studies.

Is health status linked with isolation? At the preliminary stage of analysis it was, perhaps, rather surprising that that there were no statistically significant associations demonstrated between isolation and physical or mental health or expectations regarding health status. The studies reported by Wenger et al. (1996) suggest that there is a link between isolation and health, specifically depression. Clearly further research is needed here to establish the nature of the relationship between isolation and health status. Indeed there are few studies overall looking at the factors predicting (or conferring protection) isolation as this has been studied much less than loneliness.

## Social resources

Social networks, broadly defined as availability of and contact with family, friends and neighbours, were linked at the preliminary stage of analysis with both loneliness and isolation. Different studies that have used multivariate analyses are virtually consistent in demonstrating that loneliness is not statistically associated with social networks. Only one longitudinal study (Holmen and Furukawa, 2002) has reported an association between loneliness and variables that have been used to 'measure' social networks: lack of a confiding relationship and dissatisfaction with relationships. On the other hand, social isolation has been shown to be associated with social network variables. Both our study and that reported by Wenger (1996) reinforce the importance of the confiding relationship and access to a social network (broadly defined) for isolation.

Hence these two aspects of social exclusion demonstrate quite distinctive pathways of association. Perhaps the easiest of these states to ameliorate in public policy terms would be isolation. This is clearly linked with size and nature of social linkages and developing these could, in theory at least, reduce levels of isolation. However, we need to exercise some caution in developing this argument as it is far too simplistic to see isolation in terms of contact with and availability of social networks. There is clearly an issue of relationship quality that needs to be addressed. Our interviews demonstrated how older people (and indeed the rest of the population) evaluate the importance of differing types of relationships and we need to explore this much further. Whilst we can probably identify a hierarchy of relationship 'value and quality' it is highly unlikely that we will ever be able to define an algorithm that can comprehensively evaluate relationship quality.

## Rethinking loneliness and isolation

Our study includes both quantitative and qualitative elements. As such it constitutes a classic mixed-methods approach. The participants for our qualitative interviews were identified from the survey. Whilst the two studies were undertaken in series, the qualitative interviews helped inform the analysis of the survey data by offering insights into the 'life course' elements of loneliness and, less clearly, isolation. In a cross-sectional study it is difficult to incorporate the longitudinal component. However, the interviews brought into sharp focus the importance of the 'life course' in studying and understanding loneliness and isolation. This is a perspective taken by relatively few researchers as Chapters 4 and 5 demonstrate but it is clearly an important perspective.

As with most post-positivistic empirical social research we end up categorising groups into mutually exclusive segments. In our case we were interested in looking at the experiences of later life in terms of loneliness and social isolation. Our focus was not exclusively upon the pathological; we have been as interested in the non-lonely as the lonely. The interviews highlighted the existence of at least three distinct groups with regards to loneliness: those who had 'always' been lonely; those for whom loneliness in old age was a new or increasing phenomena; and those for whom loneliness had decreased or disappeared in later life.

We adopted this conceptual framework towards the analysis of our empirical data. Given the variability of the methods of measuring loneliness and the variable nature of the follow-up in the true longitudinal studies there was a fair degree of consensus in the results from other studies. From our data we can postulate that at any one point in time the majority of older people are not lonely. A small but significant minority (5–10 per cent) will experience a reduction in levels of loneliness as they experience old age whilst a larger group, around 20–25 per cent, will experience either new onset loneliness or an increase in loneliness. In addition we have observed a group of 13–15 per cent where levels of loneliness are enduring across the life course.

Clearly this is a limited approach to establishing changes in loneliness over time and is certainly not a substitute for true longitudinal studies. However, it does enable us to offer a conceptual typology for developing a longitudinal approach to the study of both loneliness and isolation. In addition we can start to examine the characteristics of

**Table 6.2** Changes in loneliness over time: the characteristics of the key groups (%)

| | Never lonely (n = 548) | Always lonely (n = 159) | Became lonelier (n = 199) | Less lonely (n = 100) |
|---|---|---|---|---|
| Aged 85+ | 6 | 7 | 11 | 7 |
| Female | 33 | 66 | 63 | 52 |
| Lives alone | 19 | 58 | 80 | 32 |
| Widowed | 12 | 46 | 74 | 26 |
| Chronic illness | 46 | 67 | 72 | 56 |
| Severe disability rating | 18 | 22 | 37 | 24 |
| Health rated good/ excellent | 63 | 61 | 55 | 72 |
| GHQ 'case' | 10 | 19 | 40 | 10 |
| Always/often alone | 21 | 56 | 79 | 33 |

participants in our differing loneliness categories. Table 6.2 compares the differing groups in terms of key characteristics. Whilst this is a complex table to evaluate we can see the strong link between widowhood and the onset or increasing severity of loneliness in later life. The variability in terms of the composition of these differing groups only serves to emphasise the complexity of the experience of loneliness in later life and the folly of using this as a homogeneous term to describe a complex and highly variable experience.

There is even less work looking at how social isolation may change over the life course. The focus in longitudinal studies of social relationships in later life has been much more strongly focused upon social networks and from a predominantly social policy type perspective. Wenger and Burholt (2004) offer one of the few studies to have looked at this issue and offer some insights into this topic as we discussed in Chapter 5. As with loneliness they differentiated those who had a stable and enduring pattern of isolation from those with increased/decreased levels of isolation and the majority group who were not isolated. Again, we would argue that there are three distinct groups of the 'socially isolated': the persistently isolated, those where isolation is increasing and those where isolation is decreasing. There is an insufficient evidence base to examine the characteristics of these groups in any detail.

There are an array of studies, however, looking at social isolation in youth, childhood and other age groups especially as linked to the experience of chronic conditions or impairments. Examination of the definition and measurement of isolation in these studies demonstrates the variability with which isolation has been empirically measured and the tendency to use the term interchangeably with loneliness. For example, in their study of the effects of receiving a hearing dog, Guest et al. (2006) define and operationalise isolation as consisting of three factors: dependency upon others, avoiding social situations and feelings of loneliness. This is very different from the social contact approach used in our project or the social isolation measure 'knowing fewer than three people well enough to visit in their homes' used by Cheng and Vickery (2006) in their study of social isolation and stroke. The attractiveness of such concise questions are evident when contrasted with complex social contact diaries that require extensive engagement from participants or some of the standardised measures, which can be long, measure multiple constructs and may be highly negative in tone. There is a need for readers of the social isolation literature to critically evaluate the measures used and determine the degree to which such measures do (or do not) measure isolation. This is especially pressing when trying to develop an overview or synthesis of the current state of knowledge. We entirely accept that our measures focus upon contact and embeddedness of social relationships. It is clear from our qualitative work that such measures need to incorporate a dimension relating to the quality and meaning of the relationships. This is clearly an area for further work as is the development of a longitudinal and life-course perspective on the study of social isolation and exclusion (and the positive side of the concept of inclusion and engagement).

In rethinking loneliness and social isolation it is worth repeating two important points that we have developed throughout the book. First, loneliness and isolation are related but distinct aspects of the social world of older people. Hence the terms should not be used interchangeably to refer to a single concept. Second, and perhaps most importantly, these states are experienced by only a minority of older people. Even using the most expansive definitions of these concepts they are minority experiences and it is important to retain this perspective. As we discuss in the next section, loneliness and social isolation are not the norm in later life.

## The wider social world: inclusion or exclusion in later life?

The focus of research examining the social relationships and patterns of social engagement of older people have focused predominantly on the pathological. This reflects broad social policy concerns with the disadvantaged, a concern about who will 'care' for the 'excluded' and the dominance of gerontological research in the UK in the 'humanitarian' tradition. Research that has focused on informing policy so that 'something can be done' to improve the circumstances of the disadvantaged. However, this focus has served to divert our attention away from the majority of older people who do not experience the pathological states of loneliness or social isolation and who are not socially excluded. A key aim of our work has, therefore, been to recalibrate the emphasis by examining the social environment of the majority of older people and looking at patterns of social engagement alongside the more usual emphasis on exclusion.

The term 'social exclusion' is, like terms such as 'social capital', used to mean a variety of different concepts. In this book we have focused on the social engagement parameters of exclusion: civic engagement, social relationships and cultural engagement. This stance is broader than the usual focus on social relationships from the deficit model approach or a concern with social support and caring relationships. We were concerned with framing the parameters of the social world of older people and with examining their daily lives in order to provide the context for our observations. Few researchers have looked at daily life in old age and how people make sense of old age through the rhythm, patterns and activities of daily life. We revealed the complexity of such lives and the use of routine as a way of adding structure and order to lives no longer framed by the rituals and routines of work.

In terms of civic and cultural engagement our participants illustrated considerable levels of commitment to their local communities in terms of volunteering and participation in groups and organisations. The importance of such participation was richly illustrated by our qualitative interviews where participants spoke at length and passionately about their engagement in local activities. As such this serves to illustrate the important contribution older people make to their local areas. Establishing historical trends is problematic because few previous studies asked about the engagement of older people in the wider social world. Our review of the types of questions used in routine social surveys about social activities neatly illustrates the development of 'the consumer society' and the engagement of older people with more consumption-based forms of activity such visits to cultural activities and meals out: activities that did not form part of the lifestyle of the older people interviewed by Sheldon (1948) and Townsend (1957) after 1945.

Relationships with neighbours, family and friends are, for most older people, robust and enduring. Levels of contact between older people and their families and friends remains high. However, we did note the way that social relationships are enacted and maintained has developed with the universal coverage of mobile phones. Our interviews presented many examples of 'intimacy' at a distance, where long-distance, highly-valued social relationships were actively maintained via phone contact. We must, therefore, be cautious when attempting to evaluate the quality and importance of relations. Earlier studies certainly gave pre-eminence to direct face-to-face contacts. Our study shows that this simple assumption is not always correct. This, however, makes developing indices to measure the quantity and quality of relationships challenging.

## Conclusion: social relations in the future?

Both loneliness and social isolation are complex phenomena that describe aspects of the social relationships of older people. These social phenomena are contested in terms of both meaning and measurement (Rosedale, 2007). As we have demonstrated, levels of severe isolation and loneliness have remained remarkably constant over time. Indeed levels seem to be broadly similar across northern Europe, Australasia and North America. Consequently, we would argue that we are un-likely to see a vast increase in levels of loneliness and isolation in future decades. Loneliness and isolation will remain an experience that is confined to a minority of older people. It is important to retain this perspective in order to challenge the stereotypes of old age as a time of universal and inevitable social exclusion. Furthermore, where studies have examined loneliness across age groups, older people do not demonstrate the highest levels of loneliness (Lauder et al., 2006b). Taken together this evidence should robustly refute the still persistent stereotype of the inevitably of loneliness in later life.

Our study has demonstrated that the nature and conduct of social relationships in late life is both dynamic and rooted in the life history of individuals. For example, we can divide the lonely into a variety of differing subgroups: those who have always been lonely and those for whom it is a new experience; those for whom old age brings about increasing levels of loneliness and those where it decreases. We have also demonstrated how the telephone and, increasingly, the mobile phone enable families and friends to stay in touch. Clearly computers, with their ability to connect people over long (and short) distances offer the development of a new form of inter-personal communication. Web-cams, skype and social networking all offer new and evolving ways of maintaining (and developing) social contacts. They also offer, via links with assistive technology devices, opportunities to enable older people to remain living at home independently. As yet the IT-based personal relationships are still in their infancy and there is only limited research evidence available as to their acceptability to older people. However, as with telephones, such systems are going to become increasingly available and, we might speculate, more acceptable and valued ways of maintaining social relationships. Such technologies also offer opportunities to maintain relationships across the globe. There is an emerging research agenda in the UK examining ageing within minority communities within the context of an increasingly globalised world. We were unable to examine these issues but they are an obvious and important area for future research.

Social engagement is influenced by the wider social context. Health, mobility, income and access to reliable transport all constrain (or enable) the ability of older people to develop and maintain their social links. We have also demonstrated that isolation and loneliness and exclusion are problematic for some people in old age. We have shown that there are a variety of different pathways leading to loneliness and isolation in later life. Given this what is the potential for the development of interventions to either prevent the onset of loneliness and isolation or reverse these states once they are established? The evidence to support programmes that aim to foster and develop social relationships in later life is not convincing (Cattan et al., 2005a) and this is echoed in the wider 'social support interventions' literature (see the review by Hogan et al., 2002). They argue that we need to examine how and why it is that certain groups within the population lack social support (or in our case are lonely or isolated) and then to consider developing appropriate interventions. Rather than 'artificially' trying to develop social links we might be better advised to try to ameliorate the negative effects of structural factors such as income, transport problems and income on the ability of older people to maintain their existing relationships and participate fully within society.

# References

Abrams, M. (1978) *Beyond Three-Score and Ten: A First Report on a Survey of the Elderly*. Mitcham, Surrey: Age Concern.

Adams, K. B., Sanders, S. and Auth, E. A. (2004) 'Loneliness and depression in independent living retirement communities: risk and resilience factors', *Aging and Mental Health*, 8, (6), pp. 475–485.

Alpass, F. M. and Neville, S. (2003) 'Loneliness, health and depression in older males', *Aging and Mental Health*, 7, (3), pp. 212–216.

Andersson, L. (1998) 'Loneliness research and interventions: a review of the literature', *Aging and Mental Health*, 2, (4), pp. 264–274.

Andrews, G. J., Gavin, N., Begley, S. and Brodie, D. (2003) 'Assisting friendships, combating loneliness: users' views on a "befriending" scheme', *Ageing and Society*, 23, (3), pp. 349–362.

Antonucci, T. C. (1990) 'Social supports and social relationships', in Binstock, R. H. and George, L. H. (eds) *Handbook of Aging and the Social Sciences*. New York: Academic Press.

Antonucci, T. C. (2001) 'Social relations: an examination of social networks, social support, and sense of control', in Birren, J. E. and Schaie, W. (eds) *Handbook of the Psychology of Aging*. San Diego: Academic Press.

Antonucci, T. C. and Akiyama, H. (1987) 'Social networks in adult life and a preliminary examination of the Convoy Model', *Journal of Gerontology*, 42, (5), pp. 519–527.

Askham, J., Ferring, D. and Lamura, G. (2007) 'Personal relationships in later life', in Bond, J., Peace, S., Dittmann-Kohli, F. and Westerhof, G. (eds) *Ageing in Society: European Perspectives on Gerontology*. London: Sage, pp. 186–208.

Ayis, S., Gooberman-Hill, R., Ebrahim, S. and MRC Health Services Research Collaboration. (2003) 'Long-standing and limiting long-standing illness in older people: associations with chronic diseases, psychosocial and environmental factors', *Age and Ageing*, 32, (3), pp. 265–272.

Baars, J., Dannefer, D., Phillipson, C. and Walker, A. (2006) *Aging, Globalization and Inequality: The New Critical Gerontology*. Amityville, NY: Baywood Publishing.

Bajekal, M., Blane, D., Grewal, I., Karlsen, S. and Nazroo, J. (2004) 'Ethnic differences in influences on quality of life at older ages: a quantitative analysis', *Ageing and Society*, 24, (5), pp. 709–728.

Ballard, K. and Elston, M. A. (2005) 'Medicalisation: a multidimensional concept', *Social Theory and Health*, 3, (3), pp. 228–241.

Ballard, K., Elston, M. A. and Gabe, J. (2005) 'Beyond the mask: women's experiences of public and private ageing during midlife and their use of age-resisting activities', *Health*, 9, (2), pp. 169–187.

Baltes, P. B. and Baltes, M. M. (1990) *Successful Aging: Perspectives from the Behavioral Sciences*. Cambridge: Cambridge University Press.

Banks, J., Breeze, E., Lessof, C. and Nazroo, J. (eds) (2006) *Retirement, Health and Relationships of the Older Population in England: The 2004 English Longitudinal Study of Ageing (Wave 2)*. London: Institute for Fiscal Studies.

Banks, M. R. and Banks, W. A. (2002) 'The effects of animal assisted therapy on loneliness in an elderly population in long term care facilities', *Journals of Gerontology: Biological and Medical Sciences*, 57, (5), pp. 428–432.

Barg, F. K., Huss-Ashmore, R., Wittink, M. N., Murray, G. F., Bogner, H. R. and Gallo, J. J. (2006) 'A mixed-methods approach to understanding loneliness and depression in older adults', *Journal of Gerontology*, 61B, (6), pp. S329–339.

Barnes, M., Blom, A., Cox, K., Lessof, C. and Walker, A. (2006) *The Social Exclusion of Older People: Evidence from the First Wave of the English Longitudinal Study of Ageing (ELSA), Final Report*. London: Social Exclusion Unit, Office of the Deputy Prime Minister. HMSO

BBC (2004) *Health 'The Top Worry as we Age'*. Available at: http://newsvote.bbc.co.uk/mpapps/pagetools/print/news.bbc.co.uk/1/hi/uk/4043187.stm (Accessed: 28 March 2007).

Beal, C. (2006) 'Loneliness in older women: a review of the literature', *Issues in Mental Health Nursing*, 27, (7), pp. 795–813.

Bennett, T. and Watson, D. (2002) *Understanding Everday Life*. Oxford: Blackwell.

Berkman, L., Glass, T., Brissette, I. and Seeman, T. (2000) 'From social integration to health: Durkheim in the new millennium', *Social Science and Medicine*, 51, pp. 843–857.

Berkman, L. F. and Glass, T. (2000) 'Social integration, social networks, social support and health', in Berkman, L. F. and Kawachi, I. (eds) *Social Epidemiology*. New York: Oxford Press, pp. 137–173.

Bernard, M., Phillipson, C., Phillips, J. and Ogg, J. (2001) 'Continuity and change in the family and community life of older people', *Journal of Applied Gerontology*, 20, (3), pp. 259–278.

Biggs, S. (1997) 'Choosing not to be old? Masks, bodies and identity management in later life', *Ageing and Society*, 17, (5), pp. 553–570.

Biggs, S. (1999) *The Mature Imagination: Dynamics of Identity in Midlife and Beyond*. Buckingham: Open University Press.

Biggs, S., Lowenstein, A. and Hendricks, J. (eds) (2003) *The Need for Theory: Critical Approaches to Social Gerontology*. Amityville, NY: Baywood Publishing Company.

Birren, J. E. and Bengston, V. L. (1988) *Emergent Theories of Aging*. New York: Springer Publishing Co Ltd.

Blaikie, A. (1999) *Ageing and Popular Culture*. Cambridge: Cambridge University Press.

Blane, D., Higgs, P., Hyde, P. and Wiggins, R. D. (2004) 'Life course influences on quality of life in early old age', *Social Science and Medicine*, 58, (11), pp. 2171–2179.

Boldy, D., Iredell, H. and Grenade, L. (2004) 'Coping with loneliness and social isolation in later life: survey findings from Western Australia', *Annual Conference of the Australian Association of Gerontology*. Melbourne.

Bond, J. and Carstairs, V. (1982) *Services for the Elderly: A Survey of the Characteristics and Needs of a Population of 5,000 Old People. Scottish Health Service Studies No. 42*. Edinburgh: Scottish Home and Health Department.

Bond, J. and Corner, L. (2004) *Quality of Life and Older People*. Buckingham: Open University Press.

Bond, J., Peace, S., Dittmann-Kohli, F. and Westerhof, G. (eds) (2007) *Ageing in Society: European Perspectives on Gerontology*. London: Sage Publications.

Bottomore, T. B. and Rubel, M. (1965) *Karl Marx: Selected Writings in Sociology and Social Philosophy*. Harmondsworth: Penguin Books.

Bowlby, J. (1971) *Attachment and Loss, Vol. 1. Attachment.* Harmondsworth: Penguin Books.

Bowling, A. (1995) 'What things are important in people's lives? A survey of the public's judgements to inform scales of health related quality of life', *Social Science and Medicine*, 41, (10), pp. 1447–1462.

Bowling, A. (2005) *Ageing Well: Quality of Life in Old Age.* Maidenhead: Open University Press.

Bowling, A. (2006) 'Lay perceptions of successful ageing: findings from a national survey of middle aged and older adults in Britain', *European Journal of Ageing*, 3, (3), pp. 123–136.

Bowling, A., Banister, D., Sutton, S., Evans, O. and Windsor, J. (2002) 'A multidimensional model of the quality of life in older age', *Aging and Mental Health*, 6, (4), pp. 355–371.

Bowling, A. and Browne, P. D. (1991) 'Social networks, health and emotional well-being among the oldest old in London', *Journal of Gerontology*, 46, 1, pp. 520–532.

Bowling, A. and Dieppe, P. (2005) 'What is successful ageing and who should define it?' *British Medical Journal*, 331, (7531), pp. 1548–1551.

Bowling, A. P., Edelman, R. J., Leaver, J. and Hoekel, T. (1989) 'Loneliness, mobility, well-being and social support in a sample of over-85 year olds', *Personality and Individual Differences*, 10, (11), pp. 1189–1192.

Bowling, A., Farquhar, M. and Browne, P. (1991) 'Life satisfaction and associations with social networks and support variables in three samples of elderly people', *International Journal of Geriatric Psychiatry*, 6, pp. 549–566.

Bowling, A. and Iliffe, S. (2006) 'Which model of successful ageing should be used? Baseline findings from a British longitudinal survey of ageing', *Age and Ageing*, 35, (6), pp. 607–614.

Bowling, A. and Stafford, M. (2007) 'How do objective and subjective assessments of neighbourhood influence social and physical functioning in older age? Findings from a British survey of ageing', *Social Science and Medicine*, 64, (12), pp. 2533–2549.

Bridgwood, A. (2000) *People aged 65 Years and Over.* London: Office for National Statistics

Bridgwood, A., Lilly, R., Thomas, M., Bacon, J., Sykes, W. and Morris,

S. (2000) *Living in Britain: Results from the 1998 General Household Survey*. London: The Stationery Office

Briggs, A. (2001) *Michael Young: Social Entrepreneur*. Basingstoke: Palgrave.

Bukov, A., Maas, I. and Lampert, T. (2002) 'Social participation in very old age: cross-sectional and longitudinal findings from BASE', *Journal of Gerontology*, 57B, (6), pp. P510–517.

Burholt, V., Wenger, G., Lamura, G., Paulsson, C., van der Meer, M., Ferring, D. and Glueck, J. (2003) *European Study of Adult Well-Being: Comparative Report on Social Support Resources*. Report to European Commission, Brussels, Centre for Social Policy Research and Development, Institute for Medical and Social Care Research, University of Wales, Bangor. http://www.bangor.ac.uk/esaw/social%20resources%20final%20report.pdf

Cacioppo, J. T., Hughes, M. E., Waite, L. J., Hawkley, L. C. and Thisted, R. A. (2006) 'Loneliness as a specific risk factor for depressive symptoms: cross-sectional and longitudinal analyses', *Psychology and Aging*, 21, (1), pp. 140–151.

Cattan, M. and Ingold, K. (2003) 'Implementing change: the alleviation of social isolation and loneliness among older people in Leeds', *Journal of Mental Health Promotion*, 2, (3), pp. 12–19.

Cattan, M., Newell, C., Bond, J. and White, M. (2003) 'Alleviating social isolation and loneliness among older people', *International Journal of Mental Health Promotion*, 5, (3), pp. 20–30.

Cattan, M., White, M., Bond, J. and Learmonth, A. (2005a) 'Preventing social isolation and loneliness among older people: a systematic review of health promotion interventions', *Ageing and Society*, 25, pp. 41–68.

Cattan, M., White, M., Learmonth, A. and Bond, J. (2005b) 'Are services and activities for socially isolated and lonely older people accessible, equitable, and inclusive?' *Research, Policy and Planning*, 23, (3), pp. 149–164.

Chalise, H. N., Saito, T., Takahashi, M. and Kai, I. (2007) 'Relationship specialization amongst sources and receivers of social support and its correlations with loneliness and subjective well-being: a cross sectional study of Nepalese older adults', *Archives of Gerontology and Geriatrics*, 44, (3), pp. 299–314.

Charles, N., Davies, C. and Harris, C. (2003) *Family Formation and Kin*

*Relationships: 40 years of social change.* Available at: http://www.swansea.ac.uk/ssid/Research/R7H/Working%20Papers.htm.

Chen, X., He, Y., de Oliveira, A. M., Coco, A. L., Zappulla, C., Kaspar, V., Schneider, B., Valdivia, I. A., Tse, H. C. and Desouza, A. (2004) 'Loneliness and social adaptation in Brazilian, Canadian, Chinese and Italian children: a multi-national comparative study', *Journal of Child Psychology and Psychiatry*, 45, (8), pp. 1373–1384.

Cheng, E. and Vickery, B. (2006) 'Is there a relationship between prestroke social isolation and outcomes following stroke?' *Nature Clinical Practice Neurology*, 2, (1), pp. 16–17.

China Daily (2006) *Concern over Plight of Old People in Countryside* (March 9 2006). Available at: http://www.china.org.cn/english/zhuanti/country/160798.htm (Accessed: 31 August 2007).

Cicirelli, V. G. (1995) *Sibling Relationships across the Life Span*. New York: Springer.

Cohen-Mansfield, J. and Parpura-Gill, A. (2007) 'Loneliness in older persons: a theoretical model and empirical findings', *International Psychogeriatrics*, 19, (2), pp. 279–294.

Connidis, I. A. (2001) *Family Ties and Aging*. Thousand Oaks: Sage Publications.

Connidis, I. A. (2005) 'Sibling ties across time: the middle and later years', in Johnson, M., Bengtson, V. L., Coleman, P. G. and Kirkwood, T. B. L. (eds) *The Cambridge Handbook of Age and Ageing*. Cambridge: Cambridge University Press, pp. 429–436.

Connidis, I. A. (2006) 'Intimate relationships: learning from later life experience', in Calasanti, T. and Slevin, K. (eds) *Age Matters: Realigning Feminist Thinking*. New York: Routledge, pp. 123–154.

Conrad, P. and Schneider, J. W. (1980) *Deviance and Medicalisation. From Badness to Sickness*. St Louis: CV Mosby.

Cooley, C. H. (1902) *Human Nature and the Social Order*. New York: Charles Scribner.

Corner, L. (1999) 'Developing approaches to person-centred outcome measures for older people in rehabilitation settings'. Unpublished PhD thesis. University of Newcastle upon Tyne.

Cornwell, J. (1984) *Hard-earned Lives: Accounts of Health and Illness from east London*. London: Tavistock.

Cramer, K. M. and Barry, J. E. (1999) 'Conceptualizations and measures of loneliness: a comparison of subscales', *Personality and Individual Differences*, 27, (3), pp. 491–502.

Cronbach, L. J. (1951) 'Coefficient alpha and the internal structure of tests', *Psychometrika*, 16, pp. 297–334.

Cumming, E. and Henry, W. E. (1961) *Growing Old: The Process of Disengagement*. New York: Basic Books.

Cutrona, C. E. (1982) 'Transition to college: loneliness and the process of social adjustment', in Peplau, L. A. and Perlman, D. (eds) *Loneliness: a Sourcebook of Current Theory, Research and Therapy*. New York: Wiley Interscience.

Davey, J. A. (2002) 'Active ageing and education in mid and later life', *Ageing and Society*, 22, pp. 95–113.

Davey, J. A. (2007) 'Older people and transport: coping without a car', *Ageing and Society*, 27, (1), pp. 49–65.

de Jong-Gierveld, J. (1987) 'Developing and testing a model of loneliness', *Journal of Personality and Social Psychology*, 53, pp. 119–128.

de Jong-Gierveld, J. (1998) 'A review of loneliness: concept and definitions, determinants and consequences', *Reviews in Clinical Gerontology*, 8, pp. 73–100.

de Jong-Gierveld, J. and Havens, B. (2004) 'Cross-national comparisons of social isolation and loneliness: introduction and overview', *Canadian Journal on Aging / La Revue Canadienne du Vieillissement*, 23, (2), pp. 109–113.

de Jong-Gierveld, J. and Kamphuis, F. (1985) 'The development of a Rasch-type loneliness scale', *Applied Psychological Measurement*, 9, (3), pp. 289–299.

de Jong-Gierveld, J. and Raadschelders, J. (1982) 'Types of loneliness', in Peplau, L. A. and Perlman, D. (eds) *Loneliness: a Sourcebook of Current Theory, Research and Therapy*. New York: John Wiley & Sons, pp. 105–119.

de Jong-Gierveld, J. and Van Tilburg, T. (2006) 'A 6-item scale for overall, emotional, and social loneliness: confirmatory tests on survey data', *Research on Aging*, 28, (5), pp. 582–598.

Di Tommaso, E., Brannen, C. and Best, L. A. (2004) 'Measurement and validity characteristics of the short version of the social and emotional loneliness scale for adults', *Educational and Psychological Measurement*, 64, (1), pp. 99–119.

Dong, X., Simon, M. A., Gorbien, M., Percak, J. and Golden, R. (2007)

'Loneliness in older Chinese adults: a risk factor for elder mistreatment', *Journal of American Geriatric Society*, 11, pp. 1831–1835.

Drageset, J. (2004) 'The importance of activities of daily living and social contact for loneliness: a survey among residents in nursing homes', *Scandinavian Journal of Caring Sciences*, 18, (1), pp. 65–71.

Durkheim, E. (1952) *Suicide*. London: Routledge & Kegan Paul.

Dykstra, P., van Tilburg, T. and de Jong-Gierveld, J. (2006) 'Changes in older adult loneliness', *Research on Aging*, 27, (6), pp. 725–747.

Estes, C., Biggs, S. and Phillipson, C. (2003) *Social theory, social policy and Ageing: a Critical Introduction*. London: Open University Press.

Evandrou, M. and Falkingham, J. (2000) 'Looking back to look forward: lessons from four birth cohorts for ageing in the 21st century', *Population Trends*, 99, pp. 27–36.

Farquhar, M. (1994) 'Quality of life in older people', in Fitzpatrick, R. (ed.), *Advances in Medical Sociology*. Greenwich, Connecticut: JAI Press Inc, pp. 139–158.

Featherstone, M. and Hepworth, M. (1991) 'The mask of ageing and postmodern life course', in Featherstone, M., Hepworth, M. and Turner, B. S. (eds) *The Body: Social Process and Cultural Theory*. London: Sage, pp. 371–389.

Fees, B. S., Martin, P. and Poon, L. W. (1999) 'A model of loneliness in older adults', *Journal of Gerontology*, 54B, (4), pp. P231–239.

Fido, M., Gibbins, R., Hurt, C., Matthews, D. and Thomas, T. (2006) *Living in Britain: The 2005 General Household Survey*. Cardiff: SO.

Filan, S. L. and Llewellyn-Jones, R. H. (2006) 'Animal assisted therapy for dementia: a review of the literature', *International Psychogeriatrics*, 18, (94), pp. 597–611.

Finch, J. (1989) *Family Obligations and Social Change*. Cambridge: Polity Press.

Finch, J. and Groves, D. (1983) *A Labour of Love: Women, Work and Caring*. London: Routledge & Kegan Paul.

Findlay, R. A. (2003) 'Interventions to reduce social isolation amongst older people: where is the evidence?' *Ageing and Society*, 23, (5), pp. 647–658.

Flood, M. (2005) *Mapping Loneliness in Australia*. The Australian Institute, Discussion Paper No. 76.

French, J. R. P. and Raven, B. (1968) 'The Bases of Social Power', in

Cartwright, D. and Zander, A. (eds) *Group Dynamics. Research and Theory*. New York: Harper & Row, pp. 259–269.

Friedlander, D., Schellekens, J. and Cohen, R. S. (1995) 'Old-age mortality in Israel: analysis of variation and change', *Health Transition Revew*, 5, pp. 59–83.

Gabriel, Z. and Bowling, A. (2004a) 'Quality of life from the perspectives of older people', *Ageing and Society*, 24, (5), pp. 675–691.

Gabriel, Z. and Bowling, A. (2004b) 'Quality of life in older age from the perspectives of older people', in Walker, A. and Hennessy, C. H. (eds) *Growing Older: Quality of Life in Old Age*. Maidenhead: Open University Press, pp. 14–34.

Gibson, H. B. (2001) *Loneliness in Later Life*. Basingstoke: Macmillan.

Gilleard, C. and Higgs, P. (2000) *Cultures of Ageing: Self, Citizen and the Body*. Harlow: Prentice Hall.

Gilleard, C. and Higgs, P. (2002) 'The Third Age: class, cohort or generation?' *Ageing and Society*, 22, (3), pp. 369–382.

Gilleard, C. and Higgs, P. (2005) *Contexts of Ageing: Class, Cohort and Community*. Cambridge: Polity Press.

Glaser, K. (1997) 'The living arrangements of elderly people', *Reviews in Clinical Gerontology*, 7, pp. 63–72.

Glass, T. A., Mendes de Leon, C. F., Seeman, T. E. and Berkman, L. F. (1997) 'Beyond single indicators of social networks: a LISREL analysis of social ties among the elderly', *Social Science and Medicine*, 44, (10), pp. 1503–1517.

Goffman, E. (1968) *Stigma: Notes on the Management of Spoiled Identity*. Harmondsworth: Penguin Books.

Goldberg, D. and Williams, P. (1988) *A User's Guide to the General Health Questionnaire*. Windsor: NFER-Nelson Publishing Company Ltd.

Goossens, L. and Beyers, W. (2002) 'Comparing measures of childhood loneliness: internal consistency and confirmatory factor analysis', *Journal of Clinical Child and Adolescent Psychology*, 31, pp. 252–262.

Graham, H. (1983) 'Caring: a labour of love', in Finch, J. and Groves, D. (eds) *A Labour of Love: Women, Work and Caring*. London: Routledge & Kegan Paul.

Grundy, E. and Shelton, N. (2001) 'Contact between adult children and their parents in Great Britain', *Environment and Planning A*, 33, (4), pp. 685–697.

Guest, C. M., Collis, G. M. and McNicholas, J. (2006) 'Hearing dogs: a longitudinal study of the psychological and social effects on deaf and hard of hearing recipients', *Journal of Deaf Studies and Deaf Education*, 11, (2), pp. 252–261.

Hall, M. and Havens, B. (1999) *The Effect of Social Isolation and Loneliness on the Health of Older Women*. Department of Community Health Sciences, University of Manitoba. http://www.uwinnipeg.ca/admin/vh_external/pwhce/effectSocialIsolation.htm.

Harper, R. and Kelly, M. (2003) *Measuring Social Capital in the United Kingdom*. London: ONS. http://www.statistics.gov.uk/social capital (Accessed January 2004).

Harper, S. (2006) *Ageing Societies, Myths, Challenges and Opportunities*. London: Hodder Arnold.

Harrigan, M. P. (1992) 'Advantages and disadvantages of multi-generational family households: views of three generations', *Journal of Applied Gerontology*, 11, (4), pp. 457–474.

Harris, T., Cook, D. G., Victor, C., Rink, E., Mann, A. H., Shah, S., DeWilde, S. and Beighton, C. (2003) 'Predictors of depressive symptoms in older people – a survey of two general practice populations', *Age and Ageing*, 32, (5), pp. 510–518.

Hartshorne, T. S. (1993) 'Psychometric properties and confirmatory factor analysis of the UCLA loneliness scale', *Journal of Personality Assessment*, 61, pp. 182–195.

Havighurst, R. J. (1963) 'Successful ageing', in Williams, R. H., Tibbitts, C. and Donahue, W. (eds) *Processes of Ageing*. New York: Atherton, pp. 299–320.

Hawkley, L. C., Masi, C. M., Berry, J. D. and Cacioppo, J. T. (2006) 'Loneliness is a unique predictor of age-related differences in systolic blood pressure', *Psychology and Aging*, 21, (1), pp. 152–164.

Hawthorne, G. (2006) 'Measuring social isolation in older adults: development and initial validation of the Friendship Scale', *Social Indicators Research*, 77, (3), pp. 521–548.

Heinrich, L. M. and Gullone, E. (2006) 'The clinical significance of loneliness: a literature review', *Clinical Psychology Review*, 26, (6), pp. 605–718.

Help the Aged (2007) *What We Do*. Available at: http://www.help-theaged.org.uk/en-gb/WhatWeDo/ (Accessed: 28 August 2007).

Hesse, M. (1980) *Revolutions and Reconstructions in the Philosophy of Science*. Brighton: The Harvester Press.

Higgs, P. and Gilleard, C. (2006) 'Departing the margins: social class and later life in a second modernity', *Journal of Sociology*, 42, (3), pp. 219–241.

Higgs, P., Hyde, M., Arber, S., Blane, D., Breeze, E., Nazroo, J. and Wiggins, D. (2005) 'Dimensions of the inequalities in quality of life in older age', in Walker, A. (ed) *Growing Older: Understanding Quality of Life in Old Age*. Maidenhead: Open University Press, pp. 27–48.

Hogan, B. E., Linden, W. and Najarian, B. (2002) 'Social support interventions: do they work?' *Clinical Psychology Review*, 22, (3), pp. 383–442.

Holland, C., Kellaher, L., Peace, S., Scharf, T., Breeze, E., Gow, J. and Gilhooly, M. (2005) 'Getting out and about', in Walker, A. (ed) *Growing Older: Understanding Quality of Life in Old Age*. Maidenhead: Open University Press, pp. 49–63.

Holley, U. A. (2007) 'Social isolation: a practical guide for nurses assisting clients with chronic illness', *Rehabilitation Nursing*, 32, (92), pp. 51–56.

Holmen, K. and Furukawa, H. (2002) 'Loneliness, health and social network among elderly people – a follow-up study', *Archives of Gerontology and Geriatrics*, 35, (3), pp. 261–271.

Holstein, J. A. and Gubrium, J. F. (1995) *The Active Interview*. Thousand Oaks, CA: Sage.

Holstein, J. A. and Gubrium, J. F. (2000) *The Self we Live By: Narrative Identity in a Post-modern World*. Oxford: Oxford University Press.

Holstein, M. B. and Minkler, M. (2003) 'Self, society, and the "new gerontology"', *Gerontologist*, 43, (6), pp. 787–796.

Horgas, A. L., Wilms, H.-U. and Baltes, M. M. (1998) 'Daily life in very old age: everyday activities as expression of successful living', *Gerontologist*, 38, (5), pp. 556–568.

Huber, J. and Skidmore, P. (2003) *The New Old: Why Baby Boomers Won't be Pensioned Off*. London: DEMOS.

Hughes, B. (1990) 'Quality of life', in Peace, S. M. (ed.) *Researching Social Gerontology*. London: Sage, pp. 46–58.

Hughes, M. E., Waite, L. J., Hawkley, L. C. and Cacioppo, J. T. (2004) 'A short scale for measuring loneliness in large surveys; results from two population-based studies', *Research on Aging*, 26, (6), pp. 655–672.

Hunt, A. (1978) *The Elderly at Home: A Study of People Aged 65 and Over Living in the Community in England in 1976*. London: HMSO.

Iliffe, S., Kharicha, K., Harari, D., Swift, C., Gillmann, G. and Stuck, A. E. (2007) 'Health risk appraisal in older people 2: the implications for clinicians and commissioners of social isolation risk in older people', *British Journal of General Practice*, 57, (537), pp. 277–282.

Imamoglu, E. O., Küller, R., Imamoglu, V. and Küller, M. (1993) 'The social psychological worlds of Swedes and Turks in and around retirement', *Journal of Cross-Cultural Psychology*, 24, pp. 26–41.

Ipsos MORI (2000) *Poverty and Poor Health Create Isolation in Older People*. Available at: http://www.ipsos-mori.com/polls/2000/help-age2.shtml (Accessed: 28 March 2007).

Ipsos MORI (2005) *Attitudes to Growing Older*. Available at: http://www.ipsos-mori.com/polls/2005/rukba.shtml (Accessed: 28 March 2007).

Iredell, H., Grenade, L., Boldy, D., Shaw, T., Howat, P. and Morrow, R. (2003) *Coping with Loneliness and Social Isolation in Later Life: A Pilot Study*. Perth, WA: Freemasons Centre for Research into Aged Care Services, Curtin University of Technology.

Isaacs, B., Livingstone, M. and Neville, Y. (1972) *Survival of the Unfittest: A Study of Geriatric Patients in Glasgow*. London: Routledge & Kegan Paul.

Jakobsson, U. and Hallberg, I. R. (2005) 'Loneliness, fear and quality of life among elderly in Sweden: a gender perspective', *Aging Clinical and Experimental Research*, 17, (96), pp. 494–501.

Jerrome, D. (1981) 'The significance of friendship for women in later life', *Ageing and Society*, 1, (2), pp. 175–197.

Jerrome, D. (1984) 'Good company: the sociological implications of friendship', *Sociological Review*, 32, pp. 696–718.

Jerrome, D. (1993) 'Intimate Relationships', in Bond, J., Coleman, P. and Peace, S. (eds) *Ageing in Society. An Introduction to Social Gerontology*. London: Sage.

Jerrome, D. and Wenger, G. C. (1999) 'Stability and change in late-life friendships', *Ageing and Society*, 19, pp. 661–676.

Johnson, M., Bengtson, V. L., Coleman, P. G. and Kirkwood, T. B. L.

(eds) (2005) *The Cambridge Handbook of Age and Ageing*. Cambridge: Cambridge University Press.

Joia, L. C., Ruiz, T. and Donalisio, M. R. (2007) 'Life satisfaction among elderly population in the city of Botucatu, Southern Brazil', *Revista de saúde pública*, 41, (1), pp. 131–138.

Jones, D. A., Victor, C. R. and Vetter, N. J. (1985) 'The problem of loneliness in the elderly in the community: characteristics of those who are lonely and the factors related to loneliness', *Journal of the Royal College of General Practitioners*, 35, pp. 136–139.

Jones, R. L. (2006) ' "Older people" talking as if they are not older people: positioning theory as an explanation', *Journal of Aging Studies*, 20, pp. 79–91.

Jones, W. and Hebb, L. (2003) 'The experience of loneliness: objective and subjective factors', *International Scope Review*, 5, (9), pp. 41–68.

Joong-Hwan, O. (2003) 'Assessing the social bonds of elderly neighbors: the roles of length of residence, crime victimization and perceived disorder', *Sociological Inquiry*, 73, (4), pp. 490–510.

Jylhä, M. (2004) 'Old age and loneliness: cross-sectional and longitudinal analyses in the Tampere Longitudinal Study on Aging', *Canadian Journal on Aging*, 23, (2), pp. 157–168.

Jylhä, M. and Jokela, J. (1990) 'Individual experiences as cultural – a cross-cultural study on loneliness among the elderly', *Ageing and Society*, 10, (3), pp. 295–315.

Kharicha, K., Iliffe, S., Harari, D., Swift, C., Gillmann, G. and Stuck, A. E. (2007) 'Health risk appraisal in older people 1: are older people living alone an "at risk" group?' *British Journal of General Practice*, 57, (537), pp. 271–276.

Kielcot-Glaser, J., Preacher, K., MacCallum, R. C., Atkinson, C., Malarkey, W. and Glaser, R. (2003) 'Chronic stress and age-related increases in the proinflammatory cytokine Il-6', *Proceedings of the National Academy of Sciences of the United States of America*, 100, (15), pp. 9090–9095.

Killen, C. (1998) 'Loneliness: an epidemic in modern society', *Journal of Advanced Nursing*, 28, (4), pp. 762–770.

Kim, O. (1999) 'Predictors of loneliness in elderly Korean immigrant women living in the United States of America', *Journal of Advanced Nursing*, 29, (5), pp. 1082–1088.

Kutner, B., Fanshel, D., Togo, A. M. and Langner, T. S. (1956) *Five*

*Hundred over Sixty: A Community Survey on Aging.* New York: Russell Sage Foundation.

Langford, C. P. H., Bowsher, J., Maloney, J. P. and Lillis, P. P. (1997) 'Social support: a conceptual analysis', *Journal of Advanced Nursing*, 25, (1), pp. 95–100.

Lauder, W., Mummery, K., Jones, M. and Caperchione, C. (2006a) 'A comparison of health behaviours in lonely and non-lonely populations', *Psychology, Health and Medicine*, 11, (2), pp. 233–245.

Lauder, W., Mummery, K., Jones, M. and Caperchione, C. (2006b) 'A comparison of health behaviours in lonely and non-lonely populations', *Psychology, Health and Medicine*, 2, pp. 233–245.

Litwin, H. (1995) 'The social networks of elderly immigrants: an analytic typology', *Journal of Aging Studies*, 9, (2), pp. 155–174.

Litwin, H. (2001) 'Social network type and morale in old age', *Gerontologist*, 41, (4), pp. 516–524.

Litwin, H. (2003) 'The association of disability, sociodemographic background, and social network type in later life', *Journal of Aging and Health*, 15, (2), pp. 391–408.

Litwin, H. (2006) 'Social networks and self-rated health: a cross-cultural examination among older Israelis', *Journal of Aging and Health*, 18, (3), pp. 335–358.

Litwin, H. and Shiovitz-Ezra, S. (2006) 'Network type and motality risk in later life', *The Gerontologist*, 46, pp. 735–743.

Liu, L. J. and Guo, Q. (2007) 'Loneliness and health-related quality of life for the empty nest elderly in the rural area of a mountainous county in China', *Life ResOct*, 16, (8), pp. 1275–1280.

Loucks, S. (1980) 'Loneliness, affect, and self-concept: construct validity of the Bradley Loneliness Scale', *Journal of Personality Assessment*, 44, (2), pp. 142–147.

Lubben, J., Blozik, E., Gillmann, G., Iliffe, S., von Renteln Kruse, W., Beck, J. C. and Stuck, A. E. (2006) 'Performance of an abbreviated version of the Lubben Social Network Scale among three European community-dwelling older adult populations', *Gerontologist*, 46, (4), pp. 503–513.

Luken, P. and Vaughan, S. (2003) 'Living alone in old age', *Sociological Quarterly*, 44, (1), pp. 109–131.

Lunt, P. K. (1991) 'The perceived causal structure of loneliness', *Journal of Personality and Social Psychology*, 61, (1), pp. 26–34.

Mahon, N. E., Yarcheski, A., Yarcheski, T. J., Cannella, B. L. and Hanks, M. M. (2006) 'A meta-analytic study of predictors for loneliness during adolescence', *Nursing Research*, 55, (5), pp. 308–315.

Marangoni, C. and Ickes, W. (1989) 'Loneliness: a theoretical review with implications for measurement', *Journal of Social and Personal Relationships*, 6, pp. 93–128.

Marris, P. (1958) *Widows and their Families*. London: Routledge & Kegan Paul.

Marris, P. (1986) *Loss and Change*. London: Routledge & Kegan Paul.

Martinson, M. and Minkler, M. (2006) 'Civic engagement and older adults: a critical perspective', *Gerontologist*, 46, (3), pp. 318–324.

Martz, S. (1987) *When I am an Old Woman I shall Wear Purple*. Watsonville, CA: Papier-Mache Press.

Mayers, A. M., Khoo, S.-T. and Svartberg, M. (2002) 'The Existential Loneliness Questionnaire: background, development, and preliminary findings', *Journal of Clinical Psychology*, 58, (9), pp. 1183–1193.

Mayers, A. M. and Svartberg, M. (2001) 'Existential loneliness: a review of the concept, its psychosocial precipitants and psychotherapeutic implications for HIV-infected women', *British Journal of Medical Psychology*, 74, (4), pp. 539–553.

Mayers, N., Naples, N. and Nilsen, R. D. (2005) 'Existential issues and coping: a qualitative study of low-income women with HIV', *Psychology and Health*, 20, (1), pp. 93–113.

McDade, T. W., Hawkley, L. C. and Cacioppo, J. T. (2006) 'Psychosocial and behavioral predictors of inflammation in middle-aged and older adults: the Chicago Health, Aging, and Social Relations Study', *Psychosomatic Medicine*, 68, (3), pp. 376–381.

McInnis, G. J. and White, J. H. (2001) 'A phenomenological exploration of loneliness in the older adult', *Archives of Psychiatric Nursing*, 15, (3), pp. 128–139.

McIntyre, S. (1977) 'Old age as a social problem', in Dingwall, R., Health, C., Reid, M. and Stacey, M. (eds) *Health Care and Health Knowledge*. London: Croom Helm, pp. 41–63.

Mead, G., H. (1934) *Mind, Self and Society*. Chicago: The University of Chicago Press.

Moriarty, J. and Butt, J. (2004) 'Inequalities in quality of life among older people from different ethnic groups', *Ageing and Society*, 24, (5), pp. 729–753.

Moustakas, C. E. (1972) *Loneliness and love*. Englewood Cliffs, NJ: Prentice Hall.

Moustakas, C. E. and Mous, K. A. (2004) *Loneliness, Creativity and Love*. Xlibris Corp.

Mulley, G. (2007) 'Myths of ageing', *Clinical Medicine*, 7, (1), pp. 68–72.

Murphy, F. (2006) 'Loneliness: a challenge for nurses caring for older people', *Nursing Older People*, 18, (5), pp. 22–25.

National Council on the Aging (2002) *American Perceptions of Aging in the 21st Century*. Washington DC: National Council on the Aging.

Nazroo, J., Bajekal, M., Blane, D. and Grewal, I. (2004) 'Ethnic inequalities', in Walker, A. and Hennessy, C. H. (eds) *Growing Older: Quality of Life in Old Age*. Maidenhead, Berkshire: Open University Press, pp. 35–59.

Nilsson, B., Lindström, U. A. and Nåden, D. (2006) 'Is loneliness a psychological dysfunction? A literary study of the phenomenon of loneliness', *Scandinavian Journal of Caring Sciences*, 20, pp. 93–101.

Office of National Statistics (2005) *Census 2001*. Available at http://www.statistics.gov.uk/census2001/census2001.asp (Accessed: 7 November 2006).

Office of the Deputy Prime Minister (2006) *A Sure Start in Later Life: Ending Inequalities for Older People*. London: ODPM.

Ogg, J. (2003) *Living Alone in Later Life*. London: Institute of Community Studies.

Oliver, M. (1990) *The Politics of Disablement*. Basingstoke: Macmillan.

Ory, M. and Goldberg, E. (1983) 'Pet possession and well-being in elderly women', *Research on Aging*, 5, (3), pp. 389–409.

Owen, T. (2007) 'Working with socially isolated older people', *British Journal of Community Nursing*, 12, (3), pp. 115–116.

Parker, G. (1985) *With Due Care and Attention*. London: Family Policy Studies Unit.

Peace, S., Holland, C. and Kellaher, L. (2006) *Environment and Identity in Later Life*. Open University Press: Maidenhead.

Peace, S. M., Kellaher, L. and Holland, C. (2005) *Environment and Identity in Later Life*. Maidenhead: Open University Press.

Peplau, L. A., Miceli, M. and Morasch, B. (1982) 'Loneliness and self-evaluation', in Peplau, L. A. and Perlman, D. (eds) *Loneliness: A*

*Sourcebook of Current Theory, Research and Therapy*. New York: John Wiley & Sons, pp. 135–151.

Peplau, L. A. and Perlman, D. (1982) 'Perspectives on loneliness', in Peplau, L. A. and Perlman, D. (eds) *Loneliness: a Sourcebook of Current Theory, Research and Therapy*. New York: John Wiley & Sons, pp. 1–20.

Pepper, S. (1981) 'Problems in the quantification of frequency expressions', in Fiske, D. W. (ed) *New Directions for Methodology of Social and Behavioural Science: Problems with Language Imprecision*. San Francisco: Jossey-Bass, pp. 25–41.

Percival, J. (2002) 'Domestic spaces: uses and meanings in the daily lives of older people', *Ageing and Society*, 22, (6), pp. 729–749.

Perlman, D. and Peplau, L. A. (1982) 'Theoretical approaches to loneliness', in Peplau, L. A. and Perlman, D. (eds) *Loneliness: a Sourcebook of Current Theory, Research and Therapy*. New York: John Wiley & Sons, pp. 123–134.

Phillipson, C. (1997) 'Social relationships in later life: a review of the research literature', *International Journal of Geriatric Psychiatry*, 12, pp. 505–512.

Phillipson, C. (2002) *Transitions from Work to Retirement: Developing a New Social Contract*. Policy Press.

Phillipson, C. (2007) 'The "elected" and the "excluded": sociological perspectives on the experience of place and community in old age', *Ageing and Society*, 27, pp. 321–342.

Phillipson, C., Allan, G. and Morgan, D. (eds) (2004) *Social Networks and Social Exclusion: Sociological Perspectives and Policy Perspectives*. Aldershot: Ashgate Books.

Phillipson, C., Bengtson, V. and Lowenstein, A. (2003) 'From family groups to personal communities: social capital and social change in the family life of older adults', in *Global Aging and Challenges to Families*. New York: Aldine de Gruyter.

Phillipson, C., Bernard, M., Phillips, J. and Ogg, J. (1998) 'The family and community life of older people: household composition and social networks in three urban areas', *Ageing and Society*, 18, pp. 259–289.

Phillipson, C., Bernard, M., Phillips, J. and Ogg, J. (1999) 'Older people's experiences of community life: patterns of neighbouring in three urban areas', *Sociological Review*, 47, (4), pp. 715–743.

Phillipson, C., Bernard, M., Phillips, J. and Ogg, J. (2001) *The Family and Community Life of Older People*. London: Routledge.

Pierce, L. L., Wilkinson, L. K. and Anderson, J. (2003) 'Analysis of the concept of aloneness', *Journal of Gerontological Nursing*, 29, (7), pp. 20–25.

Pinder, R. and Hillier, S. (2001) 'Is there space for ethnography? Reflections on evaluating a medical student befriending scheme with elderly people', *Education and Ageing*, 16, (2), pp. 203–228.

Pinquart, M. and Sorensen, S. (2001) 'Gender differences in self-concept and psychological well-being in old age: a meta-analysis', *The Journals of Gerontology. Series B, Psychological Sciences and Social Sciences*, 56, (4), pp. 195–213.

Powell, J. L. (2005) *Social theory and Aging*. New York: Rowman and Littlefield.

Powell, J. L. (2006) *Rethinking Social Theory and Later Life*. New York: Nova Science Press.

Prince, M. J., Harwood, R. H., Blizard, R. A., Thomas, A. and Mann, A. H. (1997) 'Social support deficits, loneliness and life events as risk factors for depression in old age: The Gospel Oak Project, VI', *Psychological Medicine*, 27, (2), pp. 323–332.

Qureshi, H. and Walker, A. (1989) *The Caring Relationship. Elderly People and their Families*. London: Macmillan.

RIS MRC CFAS Resource Implications Study Group of the Medical Research Council Cognitive Function and Ageing Study (1999) 'Informal caregiving for frail older people at home and in long-term care institutions: who are the key supporters?' *Health and Social Care in the Community*, 7, (6), pp. 434–444.

Robertson, A. (1997) 'Beyond apocalyptic demography: towards a moral economy of interdependence', *Ageing and Society*, 17, pp. 425–446.

Rogers, C. R. (1970) 'The lonely person and his experiences in an encounter group', in *Carl Rogers on Encounter Groups*. New York: Harper & Row.

Rokach, A. (1990) 'Surviving and coping with loneliness', *The Journal of Psychology*, 124, (1), pp. 39–54.

Rosedale, M. (2007) 'Loneliness: an exploration of meaning', *Journal of the American Psychiatric Nurses Association*, 13, (4), pp. 201–209.

Rosser, C. and Harris, C. C. (1965) *The Family and Social Change: a*

*Study of Family and Kinship in a South Wales Town.* London: Routledge & Kegan Paul.

Routasalo, P. E., Savikko, N., Tilvis, R. S., Strandberg, T. E. and Pitkala, K. H. (2006) 'Social contacts and their relationships to loneliness among aged people – a population-based study', *Gerontology*, 52, (3), pp. 181–187.

Rowe, J. W. and Kahn, R. L. (1997) 'Successful aging', *Gerontologist*, 37, (4), pp. 433–440.

Russell, C. and Schofield, T. (1999) 'Social isolation in old age: a qualitative exploration of service providers' perceptions', *Ageing and Society*, 19, pp. 69–91.

Russell, D. (1982) 'The measurement of loneliness', in Peplau, L. A. and Perlman, D. (eds) *Loneliness: a Sourcebook of Current Theory, Research and Therapy.* New York: John Wiley & Sons, pp. 81–104.

Russell, D., Peplau, L. A. and Ferguson, M. L. (1978) 'Developing a measure of loneliness', *Journal of Personality Assessment*, 42, pp. 290–294.

Samuelsson, G., Sundstrom, G., Dehlin, O. and Hagsburg, B. (1998) 'Formal support, mental disorders and personal characteristics: a 25 year follow up', *Health and Social Care in the Community*, 11, (2), pp. 95–102.

Sand, L. and Strang, P. (2006) 'Existential loneliness in a palliative home care setting', *Journal of Palliative Medicine*, 9, (6), pp. 1376–1387.

Savikko, N., Routasalo, P., Tilvis, R. S., Strandberg, T. E. and Pitkala, K. H. (2005) 'Predictors and subjective causes of loneliness in an aged population', *Archives of Gerontology and Geriatrics*, 41, (3), pp. 223–233.

Schaeffer, N. C. (1991) 'Hardly ever or constantly? Group comparisons using vague quantifiers', *Public Opinion Quarterly*, 55, pp. 395–423.

Scharf, T. (2005) 'Recruiting older research participants: lessons from deprived neighbourhoods', in Holland, C. (ed.) *Recruitment and Sampling: Qualitative Research with Older People.* London: Centre for Policy on Ageing, pp. 29–43.

Scharf, T., Phillipson, C., Kingston, P. and Smith, A. E. (2001) 'Social exclusion and older people: exploring the connections', *Education and Ageing*, 16, (3), pp. 303–320.

Scharf, T., Phillipson, C. and Smith, A. (2005a) *Multiple Exclusion and*

*Quality of Life amongst Excluded Older People in Disadvantaged Neighbourhoods.* Social Exclusion Unit, London: Office of the Deputy Prime Minister, HMSO, March.

Scharf, T., Phillipson, C. and Smith, A. E. (2003) 'Older people's perceptions of the neighbourhood: evidence from socially deprived urban areas', *Sociological Research Online*, 8, (4), pp. 20. http://www.socresonline.org.uk/8/4/contents.html.

Scharf, T., Phillipson, C. and Smith, A. E. (2004) 'Poverty and social exclusion – growing older in deprived urban neighbourhoods', in Walker, A. and Hennessy, C. H. (eds) *Growing Older: Quality of Life in Old Age.* Maidenhead: Open University Press, pp. 81–106.

Scharf, T., Phillipson, C. and Smith, A. E. (2005b) *Multiple Exclusion and Quality of Life Amongst Excluded Older People in Disadvantaged Neighbourhoods.* London: Stationery Office: Social Exclusion Unit, Office of the Deputy Prime Minister.

Scharf, T., Phillipson, C. and Smith, A. E. (2005c) 'Poverty and social exclusion: experiences of older people from black and ethnic minority groups in deprived areas', in Walker, A. and Northmore, S. (eds) *Growing Older in a Black and Minority Ethnic Group.* London: Age Concern England, pp. 33–44.

Scharf, T., Phillipson, C. and Smith, A. E. (2005d) 'Social exclusion of older people in deprived urban communities of England', *European Journal of Ageing*, 2, (2), pp. 76–87.

Scharf, T., Phillipson, C. and Smith, A. E. (2007) 'Aging in a difficult place; assessing the impact of urban deprivation on older people', in Wahl, H.-W., Tesch-Römer, C. and Hoff, A. (eds) *New Dynamics in Old Age: Individual, Environmental and Societal Perspectives.* Amityville, NY: Baywood.

Scharf, T., Phillipson, C., Smith, A. and Kingston, P. (2002) *Growing Older in Socially Deprived Areas: Social Exclusion in Later Life.* London: Help the Aged.

Scharf, T. and Smith, A. E. (2004) 'Older people in urban neighbourhoods: addressing the risk of social exclusion in later life', in Phillipson, C., Allan, G. and Morgan, D. (eds) *Social Networks and Social Exclusion.* Aldershot: Ashgate, pp. 162–179.

Seebrooke, J. (1973) *Loneliness.* London: Maurice Temple Smith.

Seeman, T. E. and Berkman, L. F. (1988) 'Structural characteristics of social networks and their relationship with social support in the elderly: who provides support', *Social Science and Medicine*, 26, pp. 737–749.

Shanas, E., Townsend, P., Wedderburn, D., Friis, H., Milhoj, P. and Stehouwer, J. (1968) *Old People in Three Industrial Societies.* London: Routledge & Kegan Paul.

Sheldon, J. H. (1948) *The Social Medicine of Old Age.* London: Oxford University Press.

Shelton, N. and Grundy, E. (2000) 'Proximity of adult children to their parents in Great Britain', *International Journal of Population Geography*, 6, pp. 181–195.

Silva, E. and Bennet, T. (eds) (2003) *Contemporary Culture and Everyday Life.* Durham: Sociology Press.

Sinclair, D., Swan, A. and Pearson, A. (2007) *Social Inclusion and Older People.* London: Help the Aged.

Smith, A. E., Sim, J., Scharf, T. and Phillipson, C. (2004) 'Determinants of quality of life amongst older people in deprived neighbourhoods', *Ageing and Society*, 24, (5), pp. 793–814.

Solano, C. H. (1980) 'Two measures of loneliness: a comparison', *Psychological Reports*, 46, pp. 23–28.

Steed, L., Boldy, D., Grenade, L. and Iredell, H. (2007) 'The demographics of loneliness amongst older people in Perth, Western Australia', *Australiasian Journal on Ageing*, 26, (2), pp. 81–86.

Stek, M. L., Gussekloo, J., Beekman, A. T., van Tilburg, W. and Westendorp, R. G. (2004) 'Prevalence, correlates and recognition of depression in the oldest old: the Leiden 85-plus study', *Journal of Affective Disorders*, 78, (3), pp. 193–200.

Stevens, N. (2001) 'Combating loneliness: a friendship enrichment programme for older women', *Ageing and Society*, 21, (2), pp. 183–202.

Thane, P. (2000) *Old age in English History: Past Experiences, Present Issues.* Oxford: Oxford University Press.

Thompson, J. (1973) 'Adaptations to loneliness in old age', *Proceedings of the Royal Society of Medicine*, 66, (9), pp. 887.

Tiikkainen, P. and Heikkinen, R. L. (2005) 'Associations between loneliness, depressive symptoms and perceived togetherness in older people', *Aging and Mental Health*, 9, (6), pp. 526–534.

Tiikkainen, P., Heikkinen, R. L. and Leskinen, E. (2004) 'The structure and stability of perceived togetherness in elderly people during a 5-year follow-up', *Journal of Applied Gerontology*, 23, pp. 279–294.

Tijhuis, M. A. R., de Jong-Gierveld, J., Feskens, E. J. M. and Kromhout, D. (1999) 'Changes in and factors related to loneliness in older men. The Zutphen Elderly Study', *Age and Ageing*, 28, (5), pp. 491–495.

Tomaka, J., Thompson, S. and Palacios, R. (2006) 'The relation of social isolation, loneliness, and social support to disease outcomes among the elderly', *Journal of Aging and Health*, 18, (3), pp. 359–384.

Tomassini, C., Glaser, K., Wolf, D. A., Van Groenou, M. and Grundy, E. (2004) 'Living arrangements among older people: an overview of trends in Europe and the USA', *Population Trends*, 115, pp. 24–35.

Townsend, P. (1957) *The Family Life of Old People*. London: Routledge & Kegan Paul.

Townsend, P. (1962) *The Last Refuge. A Survey of Residential Institutions and Homes for the Aged in England and Wales*. London: Routledge & Kegan Paul.

Townsend, P. (1965) 'On the likelihood of admission to an institution', in Shanas, E. and Streib, G. F. (eds) *Social Structure and the Family Generational Relations*. New York: Prentice Hall Inc, pp. 163–187.

Townsend, P. (1973) 'Isolation and loneliness in the aged', in Weiss, R. (ed.) *Loneliness: the Experience of Emotional and Social Isolation*. Cambridge, MA: The MIT Press.

Townsend, P. and Tunstall, S. (1968) 'Isolation, desolation and loneliness', in Shanas, E., Townsend, P., Wedderburn, D., Friis, H., Milhoj, P. and Stehouwer, J. (eds) *Old People in Three Industrial Societies*. London: Routledge & Kegan Paul, pp. 258–287.

Treacy, P., Butler, M., Byrne, A., Drennan, J., Fealy, G., Frazer, K. and Irving, K. (2005) *Loneliness and Social Isolation among older Irish People*. Dublin: National Council on Ageing and Older People (84).

Tunstall, J. (1966) *Old and Alone. A Sociological Study of Old People*. London: Routledge & Kegan Paul.

United Nations (2005) *The Living Arrangements of Older People around the World*. New York: Department of Economic and Social Affairs/ Population Division.

Van Baarsen, B. (2002) 'Theories on coping with loss: the impact of social support and self-esteem on adjustment to emotional and social loneliness following a partner's death in later life', *Journal of Gerontology*, 57B, (1), pp. S33–S42.

Van Baarsen, B., Smit, J. H., Snijders, T. A. B. and Knipscheer, K. P. M. (1999) 'Do personal conditions and circumstances surrounding partner loss explain loneliness in newly bereaved older adults?' *Ageing and Society*, 19, pp. 441–469.

van Gelder, B. M., Tijhuis, M., Kalmijn, S., Giampaoli, S., Nissinen, A. and Kromhout, D. (2006) 'Marital status and living situation during a 5-year period are associated with a subsequent 10-year cognitive decline in older men: the FINE study', *The Journals of Gerontology. Series B, Psychological Sciences and Social Sciences*, 61, (4), pp. 213–219.

van Sonderen, E. (1990) 'Measurement of social network and social support: empirical results in relation to the Euridiss Instruments', *International Journal of Health Sciences*, 1, (3), pp. 203–213.

van Tilburg, T. and de Leeuw, E. (1991) 'Stability of scale quality under various data collection procedures: a mode comparison on the "de Jong-Gierveld Loneliness Scale"', *International Journal of Public Opinion Research*, 3, (1), pp. 69–85.

van Tilburg, T., Haravens, B. and de Jong-Gierveld, J. (2004) 'Loneliness among older adults in the Netherlands, Italy, and Canada: a multifaceted comparison', *Canadian Journal on Aging/La Revue Canadienne du Vieillissement*, 23, (2), pp. 169–180.

van Tilburg, T. G., de Jong-Gierveld, J., Lecchini, L. and Marsiglia, D. (1998) 'Social integration and loneliness: a comparative study among older adults in the Netherlands and Tuscany, Italy', *Journal of Social and Personal Relationships*, 15, (6), pp. 740–754.

Verstraten, P. F. J., Brinkmann, W. L. J. H., Stevens, N. L. and Schouten, J. S. A. G. (2005) 'Loneliness, adaptation to vision impairment, social support and depression among visually impaired elderly', *International Congress Series*, 1282, (Sept), pp. 317–321.

Victor, C. (2005) *The Social Context of Ageing*. New York: Routledge.

Victor, C., Grenade, L. and Boldy, D. (2005a) 'Measuring loneliness in later life: a comparison of differing measures', *Reviews in Clinical Gerontology*, 15, (1), pp. 63–70.

Victor, C., Scambler, S., Bond, J. and Bowling, A. (2000) 'Being alone in later life: loneliness, social isolation and living alone', *Reviews in Clinical Gerontology*, 10, pp. 407–417.

Victor, C. R., Scambler, S. J., Bowling, A. and Bond, J. (2005b) 'The prevalence of, and risk factors for, loneliness in later life: a survey of older people in Great Britain', *Ageing and Society*, 25, (3), pp. 357–376.

Victor, C. R., Scambler, S. J., Marston, L., Bond, J. and Bowling, A. (2005c) 'Older people's experiences of loneliness in the UK: does gender matter?' *Social Policy and Society*, 5, (1), pp. 27–38.

Victor, C. R., Scambler, S. J., Shah, S., Cook, D. G., Harris, T., Rink, E. and de Wilde, S. (2002) 'Has loneliness amongst older people increased? An investigation into variations between cohorts', *Ageing and Society*, 22, (5), pp. 585–597.

Victor, C. R. and Scharf, T. (2005) 'Social isolation and loneliness', in Walker, A. (ed.), *Understanding Quality of Life in Old Age*. Maidenhead: Open University Press, pp. 100–116.

Victor, C. and Yang, K. (2006) 'The prevalence of, and risk factors for, loneliness among older people in China (under theme: social support and friendship II)', *The Gerontological Society of America – 59th Annual Scientific Meeting*. Dallas, Texas, 16–20 November 2006.

Vincent, J. A., Phillipson, C. and Downs, M. (2006) *The Futures of Old Age*. London: Sage Publications.

Walker, A. (2005) *Growing Older: Understanding Quality of Life in Old Age*. Maidenhead: Open University Press.

Walker, A. and Hennessy, C. H. (2004) *Growing Older: Quality of Life in Old Age*. Maidenhead: Open University Press.

Walker, A. and Maltby, T. (1997) *Ageing Europe*. Buckingham: Open University Press.

Walker, A., O'Brien, A., Traynor, J., Fox, K., Goddard, E. and Foster, K. (2001) *Living in Britain: Results from the 2001 General Household Survey*. London: Stationary Office.

Walker, A. J., Allen, K. R. and Connidis, I. A. (2005) 'Theorizing and studying sibling ties in adulthood', in Bengtson, V. L., Acock, A. C., Allen, K. R., Dilworth-Anderson, P. and Klein, D. M. (eds) *Sourcebook of Family Theory and Research*. Thousand Oaks: Sage.

Walker, R. B. and Hiller, J. (2007) 'Places and health: a qualitative study to explore how older women living alone perceive the social and physical dimensions of their neighbourhoods', *Social Science and Medicine*, 65, (6), pp. 1154–1165.

Wang, J. J., Snyder, M. and Kaas, M. (2001) 'Stress, loneliness, and depression in Taiwanese rural community-dwelling elders', *International Journal of Nursing Studies*, 38, (3), pp. 339–347.

Weeks, D. G., Michela, J. L., Peplau, L. A. and Bragg, M. E. (1980) 'Relation between loneliness and depression: a structural equation analysis', *Journal of Personality and Social Psychology*, 39, pp. 1238–1244.

Weiss, R. S. (1973) *Loneliness: the Experience of Emotional and Social isolation*. Cambridge, MA: MIT Press.

Weiss, R. S. (1987) 'Reflections of the present state of loneliness research', *Journal of Social Behavior and Personality*, 2 [Special Issue], (2, Pt. 2), pp. 1–16.

Wenger, C. (1983) 'Loneliness: a problem of measurement', in Jerrome, D. (ed.) *Ageing in a Modern Society*. Beckenham, Kent: Croom Helm, pp. 145–167.

Wenger, G. C. (1984) *The Supportive Network: Coping with Old Age*. London: George Allen & Unwin.

Wenger, G. C. (1989) 'Support Networks in Old Age: Constructing a Typology', in Jefferys, M. (ed.) *Growing Old in the Twentieth Century*. London: Routledge, pp. 166–185.

Wenger, G. C. (1991) 'A Network Typology: from theory to practice', *Journal of Aging Studies*, 5, 2, pp. 147–162.

Wenger, G. C. (1995) 'A comparison of urban with rural support networks: Liverpool and North Wales', *Ageing and Society*, 15, pp. 59–81.

Wenger, G. C. and Burholt, V. (2004) 'Changes in levels of social isolation and loneliness among older people in a rural area – a 20-year longitudinal study', *Canadian Journal on Aging*, 23, (2), pp. 115–127.

Wenger, G. C., Davies, R., Shahtahmasebi, S. and Scott, A. (1996) 'Social isolation and loneliness in old age: review and model refinement', *Ageing and Society*, 16, (3), pp. 333–358.

Wenger, G. C. and Jefferys, M. (1989) 'Supporting networks in old age – constructing a typology', in *Ageing in the Twentieth century*. London: Routledge, pp. 166–185.

Wenger, G. C., Scott, A. and Seddon, D. (2002) 'The experience of caring for older people with dementia in a rural area: using services', *Aging and Mental Health*, 6, (1), pp. 30–38.

Wenger, G. C. and St Leger, F. (1992) 'Community structure and support network variations', *Ageing and Society*, 12, pp. 213–236.

WHO (2002) 'Active ageing: a policy framework'. Available at http://whqlibdoc.who.int/hq/2002/WHO_NMH_NPH_02.8.pdf.

Williamson, J., Stokoe, I. H., Gray, S., Fisher, M., Smith, A., McGhee, A. and Stephenson, E. (1964) 'Old people at home: their unreported needs', *The Lancet*, II, pp. 1117–1120.

Willis, G. B. (2005) *Cognitive Interviewing: A Tool for Improving Questionnaire Design*. Thousand Oaks: Sage Publications.

Wilson, R. S., Krueger, K. R., Arnold, S. E., Schneider, J. A., Kelly, J. F., Barnes, L. L., Tang, Y. and Bennett, D. A. (2007) 'Loneliness and risk of Alzheimer disease', *Archives of General Psychiatry*, 64, pp. 234–240.

Yeh, S. C. and Lo, S. K. (2004b) 'Living alone, social support, and feeling lonely among the elderly', *Social Behavior and Personality*, 32, (2), pp. 129–138.

Young, M. and Willmott, P. (1957) *Family and Kinship in east London*. London: Routledge & Kegan Paul.

Zhang, W. and Liu, G. (2007) 'Childlessness, psychological well-being, and life satisfaction among the elderly in China', *Journal of Cross-Cultural Gerontology*, 22, (2), pp. 185–203.

# Index

'chronological age is immaterial'
  as major theme of ageing 86, 90–1
church attendance 20, 114–5
  social advantages of 126
civic activities
  types of 111
civic activities 12, 20
  access to 2
  as aspect of inclusion 84
  social participation 111–3
civic engagement
  perceived as synonymous with
    volunteering 112
civil partnerships
  creation of 93
cognitive processes
  importance of 47
communication
  technology used for 100
communications technologies
  growth of 105–6
community-based activities 125–7
consumer goods 122
contact
  frequency of 18
contraception
  availability of 13
Cosin, Lionel Zelek [fl.1950s] 10
cultural activities 12, 20
  access to 2
  as aspect of inclusion 84
  social participation 111–3
  types of 111

daily life 115–27
daily living
  problems with 38
data collection 53–4
de Jong-Gierveld loneliness scale 60–
  2, 138, 148
demographic changes 13, 85
demographic characteristics
  as variable associated with
    loneliness and social isolation
    70–2
demographic factors
  affecting loneliness 150–4

Denmark
  loneliness in 135
depression
  link between loneliness and 63–4
  loneliness and 156–7
divorce 93
  increased availability of 13
Durkheim, Emil [1858–1917] 34, 49

economic prosperity
  rising levels of 14
Economic and Social Research
  Council (ERSC) GO survey 68–
  9, 148–9, 153
education
  older people entering 125–6
email 106
emergencies
  help in 108
emotional loneliness
  social loneliness distinguished 42
English Longitudinal Study of Ageing
  (ELSA) 18, 60, 84, 94, 103–4,
  110, 112
epistemological issues
  research into loneliness 51–2, 54–5
equal opportunities legislation 13
ethnic status 53
  as variable associated with
    loneliness and social isolation
    72
Europe
  surveys of loneliness in 135
European Study of Adult Well-being
  135
everyday life
  social relationships and 81–127
expectations
  changing 13–4

faith-based activities 114–5
family 13
  changing 14, 93–9
  contact with 99–104
  networks 2, 17
  reduced size of 13
  telephone contact with 100–1
family breakdown 35, 93